The Low Vision Handbook for Eyecare Professionals

Second Edition

Barbara Brown, CO, MEd

Series Editors:

Janice K. Ledford • Ken Daniels • Robert Campbell

CRC Press
Taylor & Francis Group
Boca Raton London New York

CRC Press is an imprint of the
Taylor & Francis Group, an **informa** business

First published 2007 by SLACK Incorporated

Published 2024 by CRC Press
2385 NW Executive Center Drive, Suite 320, Boca Raton FL 33431

and by CRC Press
4 Park Square, Milton Park, Abingdon, Oxon, OX14 4RN

CRC Press is an imprint of Taylor & Francis Group, LLC

Library of Congress Cataloging-in-Publication Data
Brown, Barbara
The low vision handbook for eyecare professionals / Barbara Brown. -- 2nd ed.
    p. ; cm. -- (The basic bookshelf for eyecare professionals)
Rev. ed. of: The low vision handbook / Barbara Brown. c1997.
Includes bibliographical references and index.
ISBN-13: 9781556427954 (alk. paper)
1. Low vision--Handbooks, manuals, etc. I. Brown, Barbara Low vision handbook. II. Title. III. Series.
[DNLM: 1. Vision, Low. WW 140 B877L 2007]

RE91.B75 2007
617.7'12--dc22

                                2006039686

ISBN: 9781556427954 (pbk)
ISBN: 9781003524908 (ebk)

DOI: 10.1201/9781003524908

Dedication, Second Edition

For all the low vision patients who struggle with their visual loss
and for all the dedicated practitioners and assistants who are able to listen to their patients,
think beyond the medical treatment, and do their best to help with activities of daily living.
Also for Don, Doris, Harry, and Claire.

Dedication, First Edition

For my mother, Beverly Anne Childs, and my father, Donald Arthur Brown.

Contents

Acknowledgments, Second Edition

Thanks for this second edition are due many people. The field of low vision has changed dramatically in the past decade and there are a lot of experts who helped me along the way with updating this book. Thank you specifically to Claire Rork, the librarian at the New England College of Optometry for giving me full access to the library for research. Also to Chrys Peralta at the Vision Rehabilitation Center of the Massachusetts Eye and Ear Infirmary for allowing me to visit and witness many of the new adaptive technology devices in one setting. Thanks to my friends in ophthalmology, Jill Fleming and Donna Loupe, for their advice and input. Thanks also to the many people who work for various vendors of low vision devices for updating me on the specifics of their wares and for allowing me to use professional photographs throughout the text: Mimi Berman at Independent Living Aids, Di Bolton at Clarity, David Bothner at NoIR Medical Technologies, Harpreet Cheema at Ocutech, Tim Collins at Good-Lite, L. Connell at Enhanced Vision, Ken Elkind at Kurzweil Educational Systems, Andrew Green and John Newth at CTP Coil, Jody Klager at Designs for Vision, Jessica Kremkau at Ott-Lite Technology, Karen Myers at HumanWare, and Doris Sommers at Eschenbach Optik of America. Additional thanks to Jennifer Cahill, project editor at SLACK Incorporated, who has an eagle eye for detail and whose kindness relieved all stress from the final editing of this book.

Also, thanks to my husband, Harry Castleman, for letting the computer replace him for many months, and to my daughter, Claire Castleman, who has learned to cook so I could work uninterrupted into the night.

Thanks especially to Jan Ledford for her superb editing skills and her incredible patience and steady encouragement. She has made writing this book a pleasure.

Acknowledgments, First Edition

This book is the result of 18 years of work in visual rehabilitation, low vision, and ophthalmic technology. It could not have been written without the expert early guidance and support of Purvis Ponder and Eileen Reed of Florida State University, Barbara Cassin of the University of Florida, and Malcolm Luxenburg of the Medical College of Georgia. I thank each of them for unselfishly sharing their knowledge and experience, and for nurturing my interest in low vision care.

I would also like to thank the many people who provided current information on all the topics in this book. Janet Hession and Sandy Daly from the Massachusetts Commission for the Blind and Susan Laventure from the Perkins School for the Blind were especially helpful. Dina Rosenbaum and Robert McGillivray of the Carroll Center for the Blind CABLE technology program devoted a large amount of their valuable time explaining the latest in electronic devices and computer assistive technology. Frank Lazenby and Deborah Hudson provided their photographic expertise. Jan Ledford has been a superb editor, offering just the right amount of encouragement and advice. Most importantly, Ann Stewart of the Center for the Visually Impaired in Atlanta devoted a great deal of time and dedication providing excellent suggestions, photographs, and friendship.

My husband, Harry Castleman, has been willing to share humor, encouragement, and valuable computer time while we both had concurrent publication deadlines. My delightful daughter, Claire Castleman, has given me reason to procrastinate and reason to achieve.

About the Author

Barbara Brown, CO, MEd, is an orthoptist and ophthalmic medical technologist who began her career as an orientation and mobility instructor. She has been dedicated to low vision care since 1976 and has helped to initiate low vision clinics in Augusta, GA; Jacksonville, FL; and several ophthalmology practices around Boston, MA. She has provided low vision care to patients, taught ophthalmology residents and ophthalmic technicians about low vision, and assisted in the development of the low vision section of the JCAHPO™ certification examinations. She has seen a tremendous increase of interest in low vision over the past 30 years and hopes that the next generation of ophthalmic and optometric health care providers of any capacity continue to be vitally concerned about the debilitating aspects of low vision and are able to help their patients with compassion and skill.

Ms. Brown currently teaches mathematics at a high school in the Boston area. After having several low vision students, she is learning to further appreciate the needs of low vision youth. And after becoming presbyopic herself, she is learning to further appreciate the value of magnification!

The Study Icons

The *Basic Bookshelf For Eyecare Professionals* is quality educational material designed for professionals in all branches of eyecare. Because so many of you want to expand your careers, we have made a special effort to include information needed for certification exams. When these study icons appear in the margin of a *Series* book, it is your cue that the material next to the icon is listed as a criteria item for a certification examination. Please use this key to identify the appropriate icon:

OptP	paraoptometric
OptA	paraoptometric assistant
OptT	paraoptometric technician
OphA	ophthalmic assistant
OphT	ophthalmic technician
OphMT	ophthalmic medical technologist
Srg	ophthalmic surgical assisting subspecialty
CL	contact lens registry
Optn	opticianry
RA	retinal angiographer

Note: The low vision subspecialty designation is no longer offered by JCAHPO™.

Chapter 1

Introduction to Low Vision

KEY POINTS

- Low vision is not defined by specific acuity limits. It includes any functional visual loss after the correction of refractive error and presbyopia.

- Low vision aids are defined as devices that improve the efficiency of remaining vision.

- Complete low vision care includes rehabilitation as well as optical aids.

- Assistants are extremely valuable in providing low vision care.

History of Low Vision Care

The term "low vision" was coined in the second half of the 20th century. Prior to that time, the majority of people in medical and rehabilitation communities paid little heed to the issue. They dealt with visual impairment in black and white terms; a patient was either sighted or blind. Blind patients were taught Braille and sent to schools for the blind. If any of them had residual vision, its use was discouraged in order to "save" the sight. The theory was that using the eyes could cause them further damage. These "sight saving" techniques were widely accepted practice from 1913 until 1950.

Although small efforts were being made in various settings to help those who were "partially blind," it took a world war to make substantial changes. After World War II, many military men had service-related disabilities. Enabling veterans to return to the work force despite a "partial disability" was the major thrust behind the growth of the field of low vision. The first low vision aids were fit in 1953. Our understanding of the needs specific to low vision patients has continued to improve, and since the latter part of the 20th century low vision services finally have been recognized as a significant part of patient treatment.

OphMT
OptT
Low vision generally refers to any loss of *functional vision* that persists after the correction of distance refractive error plus common age-related or surgical presbyopia. The currently accepted definition in the United States is a visual acuity of worse than the 20/40 in the better seeing eye and/or a visual field loss such that the maximum diameter of the visual field is less than 40 degrees.[1] The World Health Organization (WHO) defines low vision as vision between 20/60 and 20/400.[2] However, neither of these are legal definitions and the determination of visual impairment also varies according to the needs of each individual patient. For instance, a patient with 20/60 best corrected visual acuity (BCVA) may have a severe functional impairment. Consider Mr. Johnson who is a taxi driver and can no longer pass his driver's license renewal exam. He needs low vision assistance to maintain his profession, income, dignity, and independence. By contrast, Mrs. Thomas, an elderly woman with 20/200 BCVA, may need little or no optical intervention if she is illiterate and does not drive or work. She may do very well with her daily tasks. In just a few home visits, rehabilitation personnel may teach her organizational skills to locate desired objects more easily. She can also be taught skills to help her maneuver in the local neighborhood. With a supportive family, this may be all the rehabilitation needed in spite of a severe visual loss. Because of these unique individual differences, the interpretation of a patient's needs becomes the challenge of low vision care.

OptA
OphMT
OptT
Other terms are used interchangeably with low vision. Examples of these are "visually impaired," "partially sighted," "partially blind," "visually challenged," and "subnormal vision." Sometimes the term indicates or implies the level of visual loss such as "severely visually impaired" and "legally blind." Legal blindness is the only one of these terms that has a specific legal definition. Legal blindness is defined as BCVA of 20/200 or less in the better-seeing eye, or a visual field loss such that the maximum diameter of the visual field is 20 degrees or less (even if the measurable acuity is good). Therefore, all people who are legally blind also have low vision, but not all low vision patients are legally blind. Be careful not to interchange these terms casually. They have different implications for the patient in terms of availability of social services and tax advantages.

OphMT
"Visual efficiency" refers to an individual's functional visual ability in spite of loss. Considering a need for services based on acuity level alone does not take into account the fact that visual efficiency varies greatly among individuals. Two people with the same diagnosis and the same level of measurable acuity may meet their visual tasks in very different ways. The acuity level

may be devastating to one person and restrict his or her entire lifestyle. To another person it may be more of an inconvenience than a hardship, and he or she will develop creative ways of adapting to various situations. The use of low vision aids increases visual efficiency. Visual efficiency also depends on training, experience, intelligence level, and personality characteristics of the individual, as well as other disabilities that may interfere with normal function.

The most recent data (2002) from WHO show a decrease worldwide in visual impairment related to disease processes since its last study in 1992. However, there has been an increase in low vision related to the affects of aging. Since people are living longer than ever before, the deterioration of eyesight is becoming more prevalent. The number one cause of low vision in developed nations is age-related macular degeneration (ARMD), followed by glaucoma as a close second. (The number one cause of low vision and blindness in underdeveloped countries is cataract.)[3]

What the Patient Needs to Know

- Legal blindness is a specific term that implies one of the following:

  a. Your "best" eye cannot see any better than 20/200 while you are wearing the best correcting lens available in your glasses. (This does not mean your vision with low vision aids.)

  b. The diameter of your side vision is very small—20 degrees or less—regardless of how well you see small objects.

- Poor vision that is correctable by glasses or is better than either of these two definitions does not qualify you for federal or state services for the blind.

Providing Low Vision Services

A good low vision clinic does more than prescribe optical devices. It meets the challenges of various types of visual loss by joining with rehabilitation personnel to offer a "total package" to patients. This package consists of many parts, and if any of them are neglected the patient is not served fully. These elements include training in the use of optical aids, recommendations for non-optical devices, occupational and educational help, orientation and mobility training, and assistance with the tasks of daily living. Counseling help with the emotional and psychological aspects of adjusting to loss of vision are also paramount for both the patient and family members.

Because all of these needs must be addressed, many private practitioners shy away from offering low vision services. They may refer all patients to established low vision clinics or social service agencies and hope their needs are met there. Worst of all, they may ignore the issue altogether. None of these options is ideal. Referral to a full-service low vision clinic is the best of these choices, but has its own limitations, including the lack of these clinics in nonmetropolitan areas. Sometimes a "low vision clinic" is simply an office that will order optical aids. The rehabilitation needs of the patient may still be overlooked. Also, in this case the low vision care will be provided by someone who has no history or rapport with the patient.

Private practitioners who want to provide good low vision services should be prepared to do the following:

- Provide low vision optical evaluations themselves and make referrals to agencies that provide rehabilitation services.
- A practitioner who refers the patient to a low vision clinic instead should ascertain in advance if that clinic works closely with rehabilitation personnel. If it does not, the practitioner should be responsible for making a second referral to an agency that does provide that service.
- Discuss the issue of visual loss tactfully with the patient, honestly answering all questions about the medical diagnosis and prognosis so the patient does not hold on to false hopes or unrealistic fears.
- Refer the patient and family members to counseling services to deal with the loss of vision and its accompanying loss of independence.
- Provide regular follow-up low vision care to ascertain if there are any further needs that are not being met, in addition to addressing medical issues.

The Role of the Low Vision Assistant

The optometric or ophthalmic assistant has an important role in this process. As a low vision assistant, he or she will be responsible for coordinating referrals to the many social service agencies that provide help with adjustment to visual loss. Also, because the assistant usually spends the most time taking the patient's history and discussing personal issues, a thorough knowledge of the needs of visually impaired patients is necessary in order to ask the right questions. By understanding the complete needs of each low vision patient, assistants can act as advocates in the process of obtaining care. Follow-up care and training in the use of optical aids is of vital importance in the patient's success, and these are also skills that can be provided by the low vision assistant.

It is the intent of this book to make each step in the low vision process clear for the assistant who is going to provide the most complete care. The assistant who only needs to understand which agencies are helpful to individual patients and where to find those agencies in your area will also find this book invaluable. With very little effort it is possible for every ophthalmology or optometry office to ensure that their patients with low vision receive this full range of services. Very few low vision aids are complicated, and many social service agencies are already present in most areas to meet the needs of your patients. It is simply a matter of locating the services and understanding how to make referrals. Then the process becomes easy as well as rewarding.

In the following chapters, you will learn what you need to know to begin a low vision service in your office. Optics knowledge required for low vision care is provided first. You will also be introduced to proper and complete low vision history taking that includes social as well as medical concerns. By asking the appropriate questions in the beginning, you will know what type of low vision aids to try and when the patient may need referrals for social services. Techniques to test the visual acuity and refractive error of low vision patients are also presented. Many routine tests must be modified for patients with subnormal vision, but very little is needed in the way of specialized equipment. Optical and non-optical low vision aids, as well as electronic devices, are discussed in detail.

Rehabilitation services important to patients with a visual disability are explained. Suggestions for referrals are given, along with addresses for specific agencies and vendors. This handbook is intended as an introductory text on low vision, and the serious student is encouraged to read further on the subject. Suggested reference materials are cited at the end of each chapter, and a bibliography is provided for more detailed research. Readers should contact their state's department of blindness services for information specific to their geographic area. However, this book should provide enough detail and guidelines to allow practitioners or assistants at any level to begin providing low vision services to patients in their offices or clinics.

Helpful Web Sites

- **American Foundation for the Blind**:
  www.afb.org
- **International Society for Low Vision Research and Rehabilitation** (organization for information exchange and research):
  www.islrr.org
- **Lighthouse International** (organization for research, prevention, education, and advice):
  www.lighthouse.org/low_vision
- **Low Vision Online** (good informational site for general public on low vision):
  www.lowvisiononline.unimelb.edu.au
- **Vision Connection** (clearinghouse of information on low vision for patients and professionals)
  www.visionconnection.org

References

1. Sardegna J, Shetly S, Rutzen AR, Steidl SM. *Encyclopedia of Blindness and Vision Impairment* (2nd ed). New York, NY: Facts on File Inc; 2002.

2. Rubin GS, West SK, Munoz B, et al. A comprehensive assessment of visual impairment in a population of older Americans (the SEE study). *Invest Ophthalmol Vis Sci.* 1997;38(3):557-568.

3. World Health Organization. Fact sheet number 282. November 2004.

Chapter 2

Optical Low Vision Aids

KEY POINTS

- Optical low vision aids use magnification to enlarge retinal image size.

- Spectacles require an eye-to-print distance equal to the focal length of the lens.

- Hand magnifiers require a lens-to-print distance equal to the focal length of the lens. Distance correction should be worn when using hand magnifiers.

- Stand magnifiers require either reading correction or sufficient accommodative ability.

- Telescopes can be used by children, adults, and patients with nystagmus or visual field loss. They are the only low vision aid used at distance.

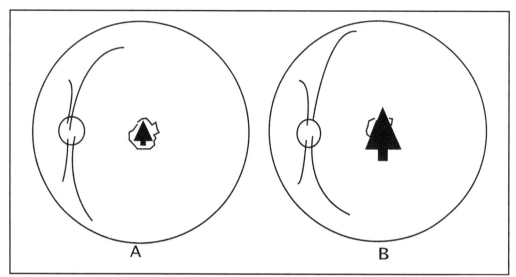

Figure 2-1. If an image of a certain size falls on a central scotoma of the same size, it will not be seen (A). If the image is doubled in size (B), enough of it can be seen to interpret the image.

Beginning low vision personnel who are not ophthalmologists or optometrists sometimes have a very rudimentary knowledge of optics. Since low vision aids deal primarily with magnification, this chapter will provide a basic primer of magnification for the reader with little background in geometric or physiologic optics. A glossary of optical terms is provided at the end of this book and may be used to further supplement understanding. Anyone actually evaluating a patient for low vision correction is encouraged to acquire a more thorough knowledge of optics than that provided here.

Magnification

The purpose of low vision aids is to enlarge the retinal image of an object. By enlarging the size of the image that is projected onto the retinal surface, it is more likely that the image will be seen by the remaining healthy tissue surrounding compromised areas. For example, a patient with macular degeneration may have a central blind area (scotoma) in the vision that measures 4 degrees in size, thereby blocking usable vision in 4 degrees of the critical central vision area (macula). It would be very difficult for this patient to see a letter that is the same size as the scotoma—a letter that subtends a 4-degree angle. Every time the patient tried to view the image it would fall on the scotoma and disappear (Figure 2-1). If the same retinal image is doubled in size it will then subtend an 8-degree angle on the retina. The same central scotoma will diminish the clarity of the image, but not eliminate it. This enlarging of retinal images is the primary goal of all optical low vision aids.

There are four types of magnification used to achieve enlargement of retinal images:
1. Relative Size Magnification

    The object actually is made larger. Examples include large-print books and enlarged numbers on telephone dial pads. There is a direct relationship of increased object size to increased retinal image size. By just doubling the size of the actual object, the retinal image size will also be doubled and easier to see. No change in optical correction is necessary except to provide focus.

2. Relative Distance Magnification

    As objects are brought closer to the eye, the retinal image size is again enlarged proportionally. A closer object takes up a larger portion of the visual field and the image will be larger on the retina. As the distance changes, the retinal image size also changes, or is "magnified," relative to that change in distance. It is then necessary to focus the image by means of lenses or accommodation.

3. Angular Magnification

    Angular magnification is a more complex type of magnification that occurs from a system of lenses such as are found in telescopes and binoculars. Divergent light rays leaving the system cause images to appear to be coming from a closer distance than the actual location of the object. The image we see is a virtual image. Our brain is aware that objects appear smaller as they get further away, so when distant objects appear larger, our brain interprets them as being closer. Either way, the retinal image is enlarged, rendering the object easier to see.

4. Projection Magnification

    Print or images may be enlarged by projection (eg, when the image on a small piece of 35-mm film is enlarged by means of a slide projector). Movie film projected to fill a movie screen and acetate sheets enlarged by an overhead projector are other examples. In low vision, closed circuit televisions (CCTVs) and other electronic magnifying devices use this type of magnification very successfully.

Diopters and Focal Distance

Knowledge of two optical principles, diopters and focal distance, are the basis of understanding the optics of all low vision aids.

Diopters

The power of a lens is measured in diopters (D). A diopter is defined as the optical power needed to focus parallel rays of light at 1 meter. Although in reality light rays are never parallel, they are *considered* to be parallel after traveling from a distance known as optical infinity (20 feet or further). So whenever we deal with optics in terms of vision, light rays from a distant object are considered to be parallel until they are affected by a lens. When light reaches the eye in parallel rays, the cornea and lens focus those rays on the retina, and we need zero diopters of extra focus power unless there is a refractive error.

If an object is *closer* than 20 feet, the light rays emanating from it are *not* parallel, but diverging (ie, spreading apart). We need a converging lens (ie, brings light rays together) to counteract the divergence so that the rays become parallel and can then be focused by the eye itself for resolution on the retina. A plus lens is convergent.

In practical terms, a 1 D lens will focus the image of an object that is 1 meter away. After the light rays from the object have traveled 1 meter, they are *diverging* 1 "negative diopter." Thus, a positive 1 D lens will *converge* the rays an equal and opposing amount, causing them to be parallel. The cornea and lens of the eye will then focus the parallel rays of the image onto the retina.

As the distance from an object to the eye is shortened, the power needed to focus an image increases in inverse proportion. Cutting the image distance in half doubles the dioptric demand. For example, at 1/2 meter there is a 2 D power requirement (1/2 meter = 2/1 D). At 1/3 meter,

Table 2-1
Distance/Diopter Chart

Distance to the Object	Power Needed to Focus Image
5.0 cm (1/20 m)	20 D
10.0 cm (1/10 m)	10 D
12.5 cm (1/8 m)	8 D
20.0 cm (1/5 m)	5 D
25.0 cm (1/4 m)	4 D
33.3 cm (1/3 m)	3 D
40.0 cm (1/2.5 m)	2.5 D
100.0 cm (1 m)	1 D
200.0 cm (2 m)	0.5 D

D = diopters

Figure 2-2. To calculate diopters if the focal distance (F) is known, divide 100 by F. To calculate the focal distance if the power of the lens (D) is known, divide 100 by D.

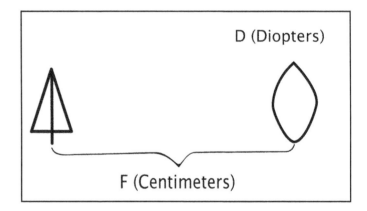

3 D are needed (1/3 meter = 3/1 D), and so on. (See Table 2-1 for more examples of dioptric requirements at various distances.) This standard principle is used when prescribing reading adds for patients with presbyopia as well as in low vision.

To calculate the power of a lens needed to focus at a particular distance, first convert that distance into centimeters, then divide 100 cm by that number. The result is the dioptric power. For example, suppose an object is at 1/2 meter. Converted to centimeters, the object is 50 cm away. Divide 100 by 50 and the result is 2 D of power needed to focus at this distance. The formula to remember is D = 100/F, where D is diopters and F is the focal length (or distance) in centimeters.

OptA Focal Length

Focal length is the distance at which a lens focuses parallel rays of light. For instance, since a 1 D lens focuses rays of light at a distance of 1 meter, 1 meter is the *focal length* of a 1 D lens. To determine focal length, divide 1 meter (100 cm) by the dioptric power of the lens (Figure 2-2). This is the inverse of the diopter formula. For example, a 5 D lens has a focal length of 20 cm (100 cm ÷ 5 D = 20 cm). In general terms, focal length refers to the distance at which a lens will make an image appear to be in focus. For example, using the above situation, the 5 D lens will focus an object that is 20 cm away, because it will cause the light rays to be parallel when they hit the eye. But that same 5 D lens will not focus the image of an object that is 10 cm or 30 cm away. The formula for focal length is $F = 100/D$, where F is the focal length measured in centimeters and D is the power of the lens measured in diopters.

"×" Notation

Retinal image size is measured in degrees, minutes, or seconds of arc, as follows: As the light rays from an object diverge and are affected by the refractive components of the eye, the image is focused on the retina. Since the retina is curved, and a sphere contains 360 degrees, a retinal image is also measured in degrees. Since the image is on a rounded surface, or arc, the measurement is referred to as degrees of arc. If the image is smaller than 1 degree, the measurement is subdivided into minutes (1/60th of a degree) or seconds (1/60th of a minute) of arc.

When discussing magnification of a retinal image, × refers to the number of times a retinal image is enlarged in size. 1× means there is no change in the size, 2× means the image is twice the original size, 3× means the image is three times the original size, etc. Therefore, if an object creates a retinal image that measures 5 minutes of arc, by introducing a 2× magnifier, the image would now measure 10 minutes of arc. This is important to consider when comparing visual field defects to image size. (For reference purposes, a 20/20 Snellen letter creates an image that measures 5 minutes of arc of the retina.)

Since retinal image size also depends on the size of the object being viewed and its distance from the eye, × notation depends on these criteria as well. Because of this, some confusion can arise. Does 2× magnification refer to the doubling of the image of an object that is 1 meter away, or double the image of an object that is 10 cm away? Since low vision providers accept 40 cm to be the standard near distance, a 1× magnifier has the power needed to focus (not enlarge) an image from an object that is 40 cm away. In diopters, the power necessary to focus at 40 cm is +2.50. A 1× lens, then, is equivalent in power to +2.50 D.

The power of a lens that can make an image appear to be twice its size is 2×. If an image is 1× at 40 cm, it would have to be moved to 20 cm (half the distance) to be viewed as twice the size. The power needed to focus at 20 cm is +5.00 D. A 2× magnifier, then, is equivalent to a 5 D lens with a focal distance of 20 cm. A 4× magnifier is the same as a 10 D lens with a focal distance of 10 cm, etc (Table 2-2).

As noted above, there is no official standard for normal, and different companies have been known to use different standards. Although most companies dealing with low vision aids have adopted the 40 cm reference distance, some manufacturers of magnifiers use 25 cm instead of 40 cm as their reference distance for labeling lenses. In that case, 1× would represent a lens that would focus at 25 cm, or a +4.00 D lens. A 2× magnifier would represent an +8.00 D lens.

Be careful, because it is possible to order a 2× lens for a patient based on satisfactory performance in the office, but when the magnifier arrives the patient may not be able to read with it. Perhaps the one you tried in the office was an +8.00 lens and the ordered one is a +5.00 lens, although they are both labeled 2×. To avoid this problem, read all magnifiers on a lensometer as they arrive in your office. Each low vision aid should be labeled according to dioptric power rather than in terms of × so the notation is standardized in your office. Once you are familiar with the standards of each company, the need to check power is no longer necessary.

Table 2-2 **Magnification Power Equivalencies**		
Magnification	Dioptric Equivalent (40 cm Reference)	Dioptric Equivalent (25 cm Reference)
1 ×	+2.50	+4.00
2 ×	+5.00	+8.00
3 ×	+7.50	+12.00
4 ×	+10.00	+16.00
5 ×	+12.50	+20.00
6 ×	+15.00	+24.00
10 ×	+25.00	+40.00

Optical Low Vision Aids

Optical low vision aids are simply magnifying lenses of various powers, sizes, and styles. They include spectacles, hand magnifiers, stand magnifiers, and loupes. Some of them have been altered from their basic style to meet the specific needs of low vision patients, but most are standard styles that are available to the general public. Please note that although each type of aid is discussed in this book along with its optics and instructions for proper use to maintain focus, it is only an introductory discussion. While these instructions are meant to be informative, it is important to know that proper training with aids is crucial to their successful use by patients. A very thorough discussion of training with all types of low vision aids, as well as specific materials that can be used with patients to teach spotting, tracking, and scanning, can be found in *The Art and Practice of Low Vision* by Paul Freeman and Randall Jose (see Bibliography at the end of the chapter). It is suggested that anyone who is going to work with patients and train them in the proper use of their magnifiers receive further training themselves about how to do so successfully.

Spectacles

Spectacles are the low vision aids that are most often prescribed, and are the aid of choice in most situations (Figure 2-3). They are simply reading glasses of a higher power than normal. These higher powers provide a shorter focal distance, resulting in relative distance magnification. Low vision spectacles can range in power from 4 D to 64 D. To clearly focus on a page of print, the reading distance should be equal to the focal length of the lenses. For example, with a 4 D lens the reading distance would be 25 cm from the eye, while in a pair of 64 D reading spectacles, the focal distance would be 1.6 cm from the eye. Stronger powers than 64 D in spectacles alone would render the reading distance closer than is humanly tolerable. The most common powers of low vision spectacles are between 4 D and 16 D.

When selecting spectacles for a patient, it is important to keep in mind the patient's refractive error. If a patient is 4 D myopic, he or she already has a "built-in" 4 D reading add. If the dioptric demand for appropriate magnification is 6 D, only the remaining 2 D needs to be provided in spectacles. The "internal" 4 D from the myopia makes up the difference. This still represents a 6 D reading *add* for this patient, and the reading distance remains 16.7 cm (100 ÷ 6 = 16.7). Do not be misled because the actual power of the glasses is only 2 D.

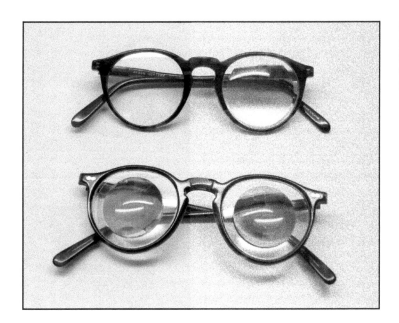

Figure 2-3. Two types of low vision spectacles: full-frame type (above) and microscopic spectacles (below).

Similarly, a patient with hyperopia must have enough plus to correct his or her hyperopia as well as the necessary reading add. For instance, a patient with 3 D of hyperopia who requires a 10 D reading add will need +13.00 spectacles for reading. This provides the 3 D needed for emmetropia, added to the 10 D needed for the near focus. In this case the reading distance remains 10 cm (100 ÷ 10 = 10).

Also include any significant astigmatic correction in either case. "Significant correction" refers to any cylinder power that makes the image subjectively clearer to the patient. If no subjective improvement is noted with cylinder correction, a spherical equivalent will suffice.

Low vision reading glasses may be prescribed as regular bifocals. This is only possible, however, in the lower powers. Although not impossible, it is very difficult to incorporate bifocal powers of higher than 6 D into a distance correction. This is because as the power of a lens increases, so does its thickness. So when the difference in thickness between the distance correction and the bifocal becomes too great the lens is cumbersome, heavy, and unattractive. In addition, the decreased focal distance inherent in these high plus adds will cause excessive convergence, and the optical centers of the near add must be closer together than is possible without the introduction of base-in prisms. Check with the most experienced optician in your area to find out the limits of the local lab. Usually it is about 4 D to 6 D. Patients who can still read with standard style bifocals are very happy because their reading habits are relatively unchanged. The only change needed is a decrease in the reading distance relative to the new focal distance of the stronger reading add. For example, suppose a patient who previously wore a 2 D bifocal power was able to hold reading material at a comfortable distance of 50 cm (approximately 21 inches). When the bifocal power is increased to 4 D, material will now have to be held at a distance of 25 cm (approximately 10.5 inches). This requires an adjustment of the patient's habits, but most are generally willing to adapt in order to continue using "normal" bifocals.

Beyond powers of 4 D to 6 D, single vision reading glasses are preferred and are often necessary. Because the reading distance is so much closer, patients have to converge excessively and no longer look through the optical centers of conventional lenses. Therefore, a base-in prism is

Figure 2-4. Half-eye prismatic reading spectacles. (Photo courtesy of Designs for Vision, Ronkonkoma, NY.)

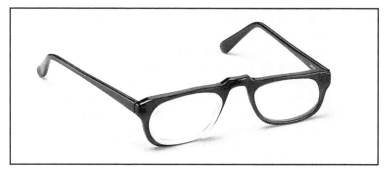

Figure 2-5. 5 D half-eye prismatic spectacles in use, maintaining a 20 cm working distance. (Photo courtesy of Eschenbach Optik of America, Ridgefield, CT.)

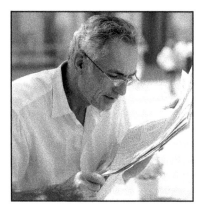

included to offset the optical centers and relieve the convergence demand. Binocular low vision reading glasses are ready-made in a variety of powers and do not have to be special ordered. These reading spectacles already have prism built-in to help with the convergence demand (Figures 2-4 and 2-5). Six diopter spectacles incorporate 8 *prism diopters* of base-in prism. (Prism diopters are a different measurement from the diopters we refer to when discussing focus.) 8 D spectacles have 10 prism diopters base-in, and 10 D glasses have 12 prism diopters base-in. These reading glasses are in the half-eye style so the patient can look above them when changing to distance viewing.

Reading spectacles with a power higher than 12 D are referred to as reading microscopes. These are usually supplied in the full-frame variety rather than as half-eyes. Low vision microscopes (or any full-frame near correction) must be removed for distance viewing.

Low vision microscopic reading glasses should be prescribed monocularly, only for the eye preferred for near vision. Since the focal distance is so close, the images seen by the other eye will be so blurred that the patient can usually ignore it easily. Also, since only one eye is being used, the patient can focus at very close distances without the need for convergence; therefore no prism is incorporated.

Occasionally a patient using a low vision microscope will be bothered by the vision from the other, noncorrected eye. In this case, the image to the nonpreferred eye can be blocked with a frosted lens or a monocular occluder. (Monocular occlusion is always an option with the lower power binocular reading spectacles as well. It is sometimes necessary when binocular viewing is difficult for the patient due to convergence or focusing problems.)

There are advantages to using spectacles as low vision aids. Primarily, people are used to them. They are comfortable, common, have no stigma attached, and adaptation is easy. Binocularity is usually maintained and the field of vision is normal. They allow both hands to be free for holding books, menus, newspapers, etc. Because they are worn on the face or can be strung on a neck chain, they are not as easily misplaced as handheld devices. Insurance sometimes covers the cost of spectacles if the patient has a vision care rider, while other types of magnifiers are rarely covered by third-party payers.

The disadvantages of spectacle use occur when higher powers are needed. The reading distance becomes abnormally close and patients find it difficult to hold material this close to their eyes. Depth of field also becomes narrower with high powers, rendering it difficult to maintain the point of focus. As the print is moved closer or further in even very small increments, the image goes out of focus. Also, holding reading material close to the face blocks available light, thereby causing shadows and diminishing contrast, thus reducing the ability to see.

When these problems become pronounced, it is time to evaluate alternative magnifiers. One option is to try telemicroscopes, sophisticated magnifying systems only prescribed by experienced low vision providers. They are spectacles that have a telescope built right into the lens. When focused for near they provide high magnification powers but allow a longer, more functional working distance. (A more complete discussion of telemicroscopes is found in the section on telescopes in this chapter.)

What the Patient Needs to Know

- When using spectacles, reading material must be held at the focusing distance of the lenses, which is *closer* to the eyes than normal. Touch the reading material to your nose and *slowly* move it away until it is in clear focus. Maintain that distance while reading.

- It may help to move reading material from side to side, keeping the eyes still, instead of scanning material in the normal way by moving your eyes from the beginning to the end of a line of print.

Patient Instruction with Spectacles

When spectacles are prescribed as low vision aids, it is necessary to inform the patient of the optical principles and the types of difficulties he or she might experience. Low vision assistants should instruct patients in several areas. The most important is reading distance. If someone is prescribed a 16 D spectacle add, his or her vision will be blurry at the previously preferred "normal" working distance. The best way to teach adaptation to short focal lengths is to have the patient touch his or her nose with the reading material, then slowly back it away until it comes into focus. Because each patient's initial reaction is to move reading material *away* to focus better, this technique is the most satisfactory. If the patient starts with the print too far away, it is very difficult for him or her to adapt to pulling it closer to focus. The patient will become frustrated and sometimes will give up trying.

The second issue is that some distortion occurs when moving the eyes from side to side. This is more pronounced in the higher power lenses. When this problem occurs, a constant and clearer image is possible if the head is kept still and the reading material itself is moved from side to side. This is a difficult adjustment to make and will require patience on the part of the instructor and the patient. Placing reading material on a movable reading stand can be very helpful.

Assistants should also discuss lighting needs with patients. Many patients have difficulty with glare or need extra light to enhance the contrast and therefore readability of material. This issue is discussed more fully in the section in the chapter on non-optical low vision aids.

Figure 2-6. A selection of hand magnifiers. (Photo courtesy of Eschenbach Optik of America, Ridgefield, CT.)

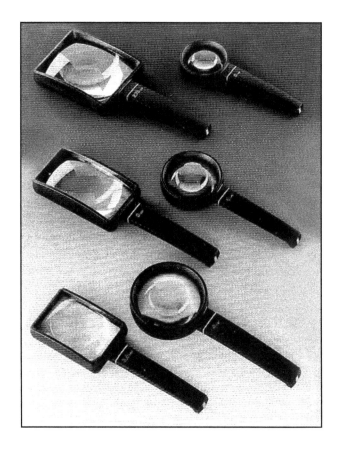

Hand Magnifiers

Hand magnifiers consist of a convex lens surrounded by a plastic or metal carrier attached to a handle (Figure 2-6). Sometimes a small lightbulb is also attached to help maintain optimal illumination of the print. Hand magnifiers are commonly prescribed for low vision patients and are readily available in most hardware and drug stores. Many patients pick them up independently to try to improve reading. The optical principles of hand magnifiers are based on the same rules as spectacles, but introduce another concept. Because the lens is not worn on the face, there is now an eye-to-magnifier distance as well as a magnifier-to-print distance.

For maximum magnification with a hand magnifier, hold the lens a distance from the reading material that is equal to the focal distance of the lens. For example, hold an 8 D magnifier 12.5 cm from the print (100 cm ÷ 8 D = 12.5 cm focal distance). Hold a 20 D magnifier 5 cm from the print (100 cm ÷ 20 D = 5 cm focal distance). This is the same calculation used to determine the reading distance for a patient wearing high power spectacles. Changing the magnifier-to-print distance will continue to provide magnification, but it will not be optimal. The image size will be smaller and resolution will diminish.

When holding the magnifier at this proper lens-to-print distance, equal to the focal length of the lens, the image viewed by the eye will maintain a constant size. Moving the eye very close to the magnifier or very far away changes neither the size nor the focus. This is because rays of light from the magnifier emerge parallel to each other (Figure 2-7). They are not converging or diverging in relation to one another, so there is no focal point on the "back" side of the lens (the side facing toward the eyes). No accommodation is needed to focus the image and no reading add is necessary on top of the patient's distance refractive correction. Patients who use hand magnifiers should view

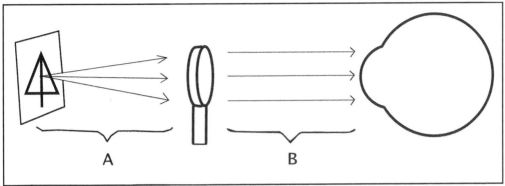

Figure 2-7. If the lens-to-object distance (A) is equal to the focal length of the lens, the emergent rays are parallel. Then the eye-to-lens distance (B) is variable.

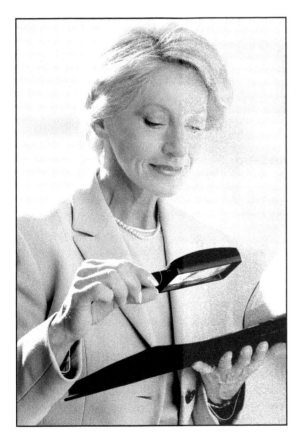

Figure 2-8. A 10 D hand magnifier in use at the correct 10 cm focal distance and correctly used without a near correction. (Photo courtesy of Eschenbach Optik of America, Ridgefield, CT.)

the image through the *distance* portion of their glasses, not through the bifocal reading portion. When using single vision lenses, they should look through the distance correction, not their reading glasses. Using a reading correction does not improve the focus or the magnification of the image (Figure 2-8). It will make both worse.

Changing the eye-to-magnifier distance does not affect focus or accommodative demand, but it can change the field of view. By moving the eye closer to the lens, the field will increase in size. This technique allows more words to be seen without moving the lens. Patients who constantly

Figure 2-9. A hand magnifier has many helpful uses in the home.

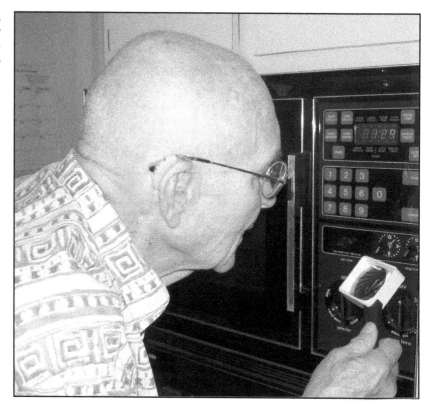

bring the magnifier to the eye for a larger field of view must be reminded about keeping the lens-to-print distance constant. In other words, they must bring the reading material closer to the eye at the same rate in which they bring the magnifier closer. They may eventually prefer a spectacle correction or loupe instead, as these lenses are already designed to be held at the plane of the eye.

Hand magnifiers are excellent for situations when the near material is at a fixed distance and cannot be brought closer to the eye. For instance, in a grocery store a magnifier can be used to look at labels of cans on the top shelf. Looking at temperature dials on a hot stove (Figure 2-9) or viewing a seam while machine sewing are other excellent uses. Hand magnifiers are extremely portable, so they are useful in any situation that requires a quick look. Reading price tags while shopping, looking up phone numbers in the telephone directory, and looking at photographs of the grandchildren are all good examples. The magnifier can be retrieved from a pocket or purse and returned just as quickly. A magnifier also can be used for long-term reading, but most patients find it difficult to handhold them at the correct focal distance for long periods. Because one must hold the aid, it is difficult to hold a book *and* turn pages with the other hand. A reading stand is often necessary.

The necessity of maintaining a constant magnifier-to-print distance is the biggest disadvantage of hand magnifiers. Patients who lack arm strength or those with hand tremors find them difficult to use. Many patients inadvertently move the aid further from or closer to the page, with a subsequent loss of image clarity and magnification. Also, the hand that holds the lens and the lens carrier itself create shadows on the printed page and block out available light. This problem is exacerbated as the power increases and the magnifier-to-print distance is reduced.

Hand magnifiers come in many style variations for specific uses. These are mostly designed to eliminate some of the aforementioned disadvantages. One type hangs on a neckstrap and has a chest support to allow both hands freedom of movement for sewing or crafts. Another type is a large rectangular lens supported on a reading lamp so a book can be held beneath it and the light kept constant. Some are in small leather cases that flip open and can easily be carried in a pocket. There is probably a hand magnifier for most any use and of any power your patient desires.

What the Patient Needs to Know

- The distance from a hand magnifier to the printed page must be kept constant. To find this distance, start with the lens on the page and *slowly* pull it away from the print until optimal focus is reached.

- Hand magnifiers should be used with *distance* glasses.

- If the magnifier is brought closer to your eye to increase the field of view, bring the reading material closer as well. The distance from print to lens must always be kept constant to maintain focus.

Patient Instruction with Hand Magnifiers

When patients begin to use hand magnifiers, the tendency is to hold the lens up to the eye and look through it. Since viewing through lenses at the level of the eye has always been normal, it is hard to adjust to a new technique where the magnifier must be held near the page instead. To make it clear, have your patients start with the magnifier flat on the page. They should then raise it slowly until maximum magnification is achieved. Have them repeat this process several times until they are familiar with the correct focal distance. Frequently repeat the idea of keeping this distance constant. Only after it is clear should you begin a discussion of field of view and changing the eye-to-magnifier distance. Patients easily confuse the two concepts.

Reinforce the fact that distance glasses should be worn while using hand magnifiers. Elderly patients are used to thinking in terms of using bifocals for near work. Some have a hard time understanding why the need for a bifocal is suddenly eliminated. (Some of them will hold the magnifier closer to the print and use their bifocal anyway.)

When discussing lighting, recommend a style of lamp that can be positioned to direct light onto the paper *underneath* the lens. Magnifiers with built-in light sources are a good way to eliminate shadows and are preferred by many people over the non-illuminated variety.

Unlike spectacles, hand magnifiers can easily be moved across a line of print without distortion. It is not necessary to move the book beneath the lens. In some inexpensive models there is distortion around the periphery of the lens. Aspheric magnifiers eliminate this problem by changing the power as the glass recedes away from the optical center. This manufacturing technique provides a clear focus across the entire lens. Most magnifiers offered by low vision suppliers are aspheric, so distortion is minimal.

Stand Magnifiers

Stand magnifiers are similar to hand magnifiers. They consist of a convex lens which is usually surrounded by a plastic or metal carrier (Figures 2-10 and 2-11). Instead of a handle, however,

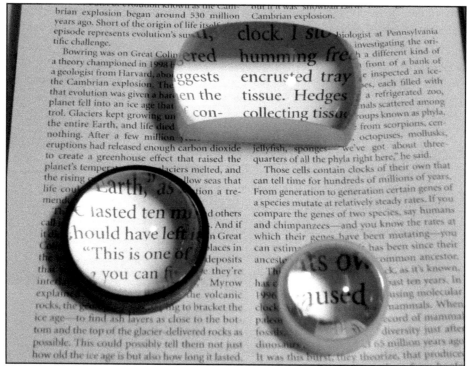

Figure 2-10. Bright field stand magnifiers sit right on a page of print and direct ambient light onto the page, providing increased natural illumination of the print.

Figure 2-11. CTP Coil stand magnifiers provide a space for illumination to be angled directly on the print without shadow. (Photo courtesy of CTP Coil, Slough, Berkshire, UK.)

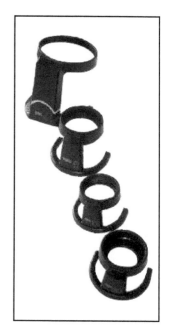

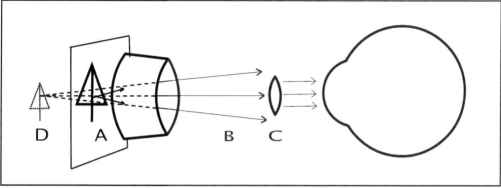

Figure 2-12. Light rays diverge as they leave an object (A). The lens of a stand magnifier provides enough converging power to counteract some of the divergence, but the rays continue to diverge a bit after they pass through the lens (B). A plus power (convergent) spectacle lens is then required to counteract the remaining divergence. After the rays leave the spectacle lens (C), they emerge parallel for viewing by the eye. The power of the spectacle lens depends on the imaginary focal distance of the virtual image (D) which in turn is dependent on the height of the stand magnifier.

they are attached to legs or some other support. These enable the magnifier to stand freely on a page of print. Some have an internal light source. Others have no carrier, but sit directly on the page like a paperweight.

The legs of most stand magnifiers are shorter than the focal length of the lens to provide portability and a clear image to the periphery of the lens. As a result, image rays emerging from the back of the lens are not parallel. They are still somewhat divergent, making the image appear to come from a point further away than the actual location (a virtual image). Before viewing by the eye, these divergent rays must be focused. This can be accomplished by using accommodation or by viewing through reading glasses or the reading segment of a bifocal. The bifocal power should be determined for the focal distance of the virtual image (Figure 2-12). Because this virtual image is farther away than the actual image, the effective magnification is less. Stand magnifiers do not achieve maximum magnification from the power of their lenses. This means that the power listed in catalogues is not equivalent to the actual magnification provided by the lens. For this reason, a higher power of stand magnifier will be necessary to achieve the same level of reading comfort as a lower power hand magnifier or spectacles.

With stand magnifiers, the magnifier-to-print distance is constantly maintained by the legs of the apparatus. It is not necessary for the patient to worry about controlling focal length, so many patients prefer stand rather than hand magnifiers. Elderly patients adapt more easily because bifocals or reading glasses are worn. It is a familiar situation for near vision and few habits need to be changed.

The eye-to-lens distance must be fairly constant and depends on the power of the bifocal. Stronger reading adds allow closer working distances and provide somewhat higher magnification. These distances are much less variable than a hand magnifier and the field of view can be only minimally improved by moving nearer to the lens. The image will simply go out of focus unless a stronger reading add is employed.

One disadvantage of stand magnifiers is lack of portability. Many are small enough to be carried in a purse but not a pocket, as most styles do not fold or collapse. They can be cumbersome and rarely have cases, so the lens can scratch easily. The patient is better served using one on a desk or table. A supplementary hand magnifier for use outside the home is usually necessary.

Figure 2-13. Illuminated stand magnifiers have interchangeable handles to adjust the light level. Some also include line guides for orientation on the page. (Photo courtesy of Eschenbach Optik of America, Ridgefield, CT.)

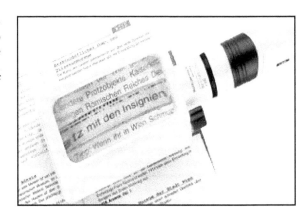

Stand magnifiers with plastic housings can also limit the amount of light that falls on the reading material. Because the lens sits very close to the page, a shadow is often cast directly on the print. The support stand itself blocks light from entering at the sides, and the light that comes directly through the lens is focused, creating a spot of light smaller than the field of view. The resultant brightness and shadow creates an intriguing test of patience and ingenuity to read or maneuver a light source through the legs and onto the print without causing glare.

Designers have tried many ways to solve this problem. Some stand magnifiers are attached to flashlights or other light sources. Sometimes these light sources have interchangeable handles which provide different levels of illumination so the optimum brightness can be chosen by the user (Figure 2-13). Other stand magnifiers have angled lenses or wider spaces between the legs to allow more light to enter. The paperweight style of stand magnifier is referred to as a bright field magnifier because the lens actually collects ambient light and provides natural illumination to the printed material.

What the Patient Needs to Know

- Wear your bifocals, reading glasses, or other near correction when using a stand magnifier. You will feel a "pull" on your eyes if you try to use the portion of your glasses that is for driving and watching television.
- Always keep the distance from your eyes to the magnifier constant. Do not pull the magnifier up to your eye or the focus will be lost.

Reading a book with a stand magnifier can be difficult because the binding sometimes prevents moving the magnifier all the way to the end of the print on the left-facing page or the beginning of the print on the right-facing page. Most stand magnifiers also have a relatively limited field of view. For all these reasons, stand magnifiers are best used for reading materials such as a newspaper on a flat surface or for reading articles that are relatively short. They are also well suited to hobbies. *Spotting*, which is looking at a subject in one location, is more suited to stand magnifiers than long-term reading, where the magnifier must be moved across lines and columns of print. Movement of a magnifier during use is referred to as *scanning*.

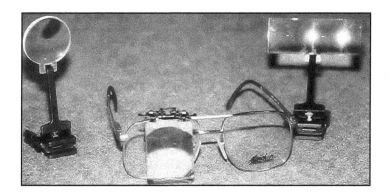

Figure 2-14. Loupes of high powers attach to regular spectacles and can be used for very close work on an intermittent basis.

Patient Instruction with Stand Magnifiers

Patients with tremors or lack of arm control enjoy stand magnifiers because the lens-to-print distance is constantly provided by the stand itself. Older patients require very little instruction in spectacle correction because reading glasses are used. This is normal and acceptable to most patients.

The eye-to-lens distance causes some difficulty and requires explanation. Patients like to pull stand magnifiers up to their eyes as if viewing through a telescope. This will improve the field of view only minimally, and blur the image if accommodation is inadequate. Instruct your patients to maintain an appropriate reading distance. The ideal length is slightly shorter than the focal length of the bifocal. If your patient is a young person with high accommodative reserves, closer distances are acceptable. If a patient persists in holding a stand magnifier close to the eye, suggest high power spectacles instead. They achieve the same purpose, keep the hands free, and allow a larger field of view.

The more creative you are, the more you will be able to help your patients with the lighting dilemma. A gooseneck or movable arm lamp is mandatory to shine light on the print yet underneath the lens. Some low vision providers remove one or more of the legs of the stand magnifier, allowing a larger window for the light to enter. Removing legs in this way also helps with the problem of the bookbinding impeding movement of the lens to the end of the print. It is tricky to provide larger light openings while maintaining stability of the base. The design of CTP Coil (Slough, Berkshire, UK) brand magnifiers has been altered to reduce this problem by removing one edge of the base (see Figure 2-11).

What the Patient Needs to Know

- Clean the lenses of low vision aids with a soft cloth and lens cleaning solution or water.

- Store lenses in their cases or wrapped in a soft cloth, as they tend to scratch very easily.

Loupes

Loupes are high plus (convex) lenses that are handheld close to the eye, worn on the head, or attach directly to existing spectacles (Figure 2-14). Sometimes they have a carrier that slides over or clips on the glasses, such as a jeweler's loupe. Other loupes are on a hinged arm that attaches

Figure 2-15. Handheld telescopes are very portable and can be used for short-term distance viewing. They are handy for use in the classroom or as mobility aids to help with spot reading of signs or addresses.

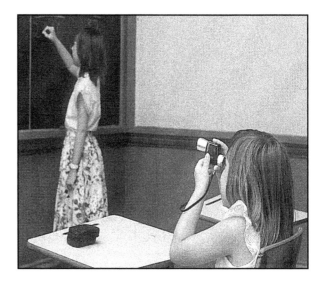

to the temple or nosepiece of the spectacle frames. The loupe is lowered in front of the eye when additional power is needed. When it is no longer needed it is flipped out of the visual axis.

Loupes are used in the same way as high power spectacles. They require a short eye-to-print distance that shortens as the power increases. The convenient aspect of a loupe is the ability to attach or detach it at will. They are handy, lightweight, and available in many strengths. They are best when used for very close viewing, as in examining photographs, coins, or other small objects.

The disadvantages of loupes are the short working distance and a reduced field of view through the small diameter lenses. Spectacle attachments usually are less than ideal as well. The clip-on types tend to slip off center, and the movable-arm types break easily. Also, as they only attach to one lens, the glasses may sit at a cockeyed angle and require more frequent adjustments. Varieties worn on the head are much more stable, but more bulky. Be sure to add the power of any reading glasses the patient uses to that of the loupe when determining focal distance.

Patient Instruction with Loupes

Patients should be taught how to clean the lenses (with water or lens cleaner only), how to store them (in a soft cloth or box), and how to attach them to spectacles. The eye-to-print distance must be kept constant in the same way as with spectacles.

Telescopes

Handheld

Telescopes (Figure 2-15) are more complex optical systems that consist of two lenses separated by a short distance in a metal tube. Astronomical telescopes are the kind commonly used to view stars and planets. Their optics cause the image to be viewed upside down and are thus impractical for other uses. Galilean telescopes allow the image to be viewed upright, so they are the type most often used for low vision. In Galilean telescopes, a concave lens nearest the eye is called the *ocular* and a convex lens closer to the object being viewed is the *objective*. Sometimes a prism and mirror are incorporated in the carrier to decrease the distance between the lenses and render the telescope easier to hold in one hand. Keplerian telescopes are also used in low vision.

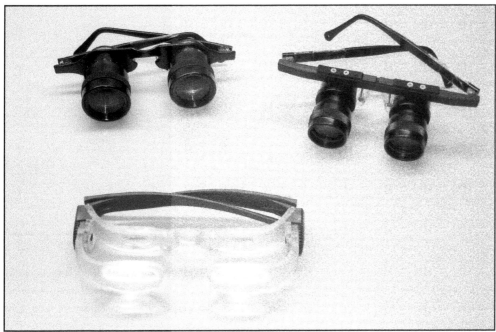

Figure 2-16. Binocular telescopic spectacles and sports scopes allow hands-free distance use for watching lectures, sporting events, plays, or concerts.

These are similar to Galilean telescopes except the ocular and objective lenses are both convex. This creates an upside-down image which must be compensated by the use of an internal prism, but it also provides for a larger field of view than the Galilean type. Low vision telescopes can be focused for distances as short as 2 to 3 feet, but most are for viewing objects across the room or at optical infinity. Telescopes are the only non-electronic low vision aid that can be used to improve distance viewing.

Telescopes are labeled according to power and field of view. An 8 × 20, 7.5 monocular telescope indicates the following: The image seen through the telescope is 8 times larger than normal, or 8×. The objective lens is 20 mm in diameter, and the field of view is 7.5 degrees through a normal size pupil.

Telescopes provide a clear view at distance by means of angular magnification. Angular magnification is a compound lens system which creates a larger image on the retina, resulting in improved vision. Telescopes "trick" the brain because we know from experience that when we view an object in the distance the image is smaller, and when we are closer to an object it appears larger. Since the image from a telescope is larger, the brain interprets the object as being *closer*, rather than as a larger, distant object. This is one reason why it is very difficult (or impossible!) to walk while looking through a telescope. Whether it is the image of the object which is larger or the object is perceived to be closer, the result is the same—increased clarity of the distant object because of an enlarged retinal image.

Telescopes have several shortcomings. As an image is viewed, there is a decrease in the amount of transmitted light, so the image will appear darker. Also, as the power increases, field of view decreases dramatically. This decrease in visual field allows the viewer to see only a small central portion of the distant world at one time, a definite drawback. A larger field of view is possible with binoculars instead of a monocular telescope (Figure 2-16). As with common

Figure 2-17. Bioptic telescopic lenses for distance use, such as for driving. The carrier lens holds the regular distance prescription. The telescopic lenses are placed above the optical axis so the head can be tipped down to view through them for spot checking. (Photo courtesy of Designs for Vision, Ronkonkoma, NY.)

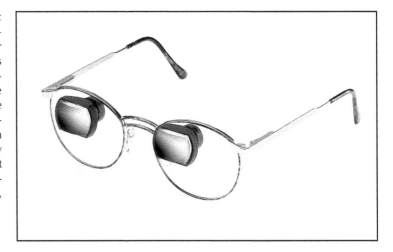

astronomical telescopes, the traditional type of binocular is not used in low vision. (Regular field glasses are too large, cumbersome, and heavy to be used for the everyday needs of the low vision patient.) Some low power binoculars are designed to be worn as regular glasses, so are relatively manageable. In this case, the viewing lenses are incorporated right into the spectacle frame. The CTP Coil Spectacle Binocular™ and Selsi Sport Spectacles™ (Midland Park, NJ) are two popular spectacle binoculars. Eschenbach Optik of America (Ridgefield, CT) makes a version as well that is slightly less cumbersome and lighter weight and can be ordered for distance or for near use. The only differences between the two are the power and the position of the optical centers, allowing for convergence at near.

If a telescope is moved even slightly, the movement of the viewed image is magnified. A 5-degree movement of the user's hand is small, but the image will make a fast sweeping movement completely out of the small field of view. This is referred to as *motion parallax* and creates difficulty in using handheld telescopes. It completely eliminates the use of a telescope while walking, driving, or otherwise moving. Arm fatigue and tremors also cause problems using handheld telescopes, so the weight of each type should be considered.

Bioptics

Bioptics are another spectacle-mounted alternative to the handheld variety of telescopes. These attach directly to spectacle lenses *above* the optical axis (Figure 2-17). The chin can be dipped down slightly, allowing the user to spot an object through the telescope, then walk toward it with the head erect looking through the spectacle carrier lens as usual. Bioptics are excellent for mobility purposes. The telescope is used to sight bus numbers or street signs, but the glasses are used for safe walking with a wide field of view.

It is legal in at least 31 states and in Washington, DC for people with moderate vision loss to drive using bioptic telescopes. The criteria for licensing varies in each state, but there are some general standards. In all but six of the states, the user must achieve 20/40 acuity through the bioptic. In no states are patients allowed to drive with bioptics if their regular BCVA falls below the 20/200 level or with a usable visual field of 20 degrees or less, and in most states it must be better than that.

Driving with bioptics has been controversial for many years. Opponents of the practice cite the small visual field visible through the telescope, telescopic parallax, difficulty using car mirrors while driving, and the need for critical adjustment of the lenses as reasons to question the safety of driving with bioptics. The proponents, however, cite the excellent functional ability of

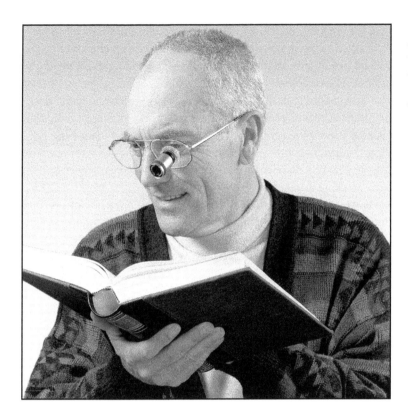

Figure 2-18. Telemicroscopes are bioptics for near use. (Photo courtesy of Eschenbach Optik of America, Ridgefield, CT.)

patients while using bioptics. The decision is a very individual one for the driver and for each state legislature. Check with your local bureau of licensing for regulations in your state. The web site of the Bioptic Driving Network (www.biopticdriving.org) is a good resource for up-to-date information on bioptics and the driving controversy.

What the Patient Needs to Know

- Telescopes must be balanced and held steady by resting your hand against your face and your arm against your body or other support.

- To locate an object, first view it with your naked eye before lifting the telescope and spotting through it.

- Do not walk or move when viewing through a telescope.

- Objects seen through a telescope appear to be closer than they are.

Telemicroscopes

Telemicroscopes are telescopes mounted just *under* the optical center of the spectacle lens like a protruding bifocal. These systems are used for reading instead of for distance viewing (Figure 2-18). A small cap with a low power lens is attached to the objective to allow clear focus at a normal reading distance. The telescope provides the magnification, and the power of the reading cap determines the reading distance. For example, a +2.00 cap focuses at 50 cm. The depth of focus is decreased in telemicroscopes so the viewing distance must be critically maintained.

Telemicroscopes are ideal for school or desk work. The telescope alone can be used to see a chalkboard, clock, or overhead projector by tipping the chin up. Snapping the reading cap in place changes the focus to desk length for ease in taking notes or long-term reading. Students in the higher grades and college find telemicroscopes very helpful. Telemicroscopes have a number of successful vocational uses for occupations requiring long-term near work with an extended working distance, such as cash registers, accounting ledgers, or other desk work. They are also helpful with the middle distance necessary to view a computer screen. However, many times large-print magnification programs allow computer access without a near aid. (See Chapter 4 for more on computer accessibility.) Patients who rely on telemicroscopes may have different power reading caps for uses requiring several working distances.

High minus contact lenses worn under a high plus reading glass can provide patients with a makeshift full-field telescope. This is an option for the very motivated patient who is able to adjust to constant use of a telescope by one eye, ignoring its use when reading or walking.

Handheld telescopes should be provided to nearly every low vision patient. Even the patient with few low vision needs should receive some help with distance viewing. The simpler brands and lower powers are relatively inexpensive, so handheld telescopes are excellent for young children who may require frequent replacement of them from loss or damage. This encourages the child to adapt to the use of a telescope at a young age before peer pressure or teasing might decrease self-confidence and preclude the use of an obvious distance aid. Most children love telescopes for television watching and "spying" out the window. They are ideal for use in school.

Since the eyes of patients with nystagmus are in constant motion, many people think they would not be candidates for the use of a telescope. In most cases this is not true and patients with nystagmus are often very successful telescope users. Very few patients with nystagmus experience oscillopsia (the apparent motion of objects). Most can see well as the eye passes the telescope's ocular lens. Moreover, most patients with nystagmus have a null point where the eye movement is minimal. Keeping the eyes in the null position allows better visual acuity, so it is second nature to most people with nystagmus. If the telescope is used with the eyes in this position it can be extremely successful.

Telescopes have another use for patients with very narrow visual fields. If the telescope is turned around backwards and the user views through the objective lens, the image is minified. This allows more visual information to fit within the limits of a patient's small field of view. For this technique to be successfully employed, the patient's acuity must be good enough to resolve the minified image. This is often the case when the visual field loss is due to glaucoma or retinitis pigmentosa, and so should be tried with those patients.

Patient Instruction with Telescopes

Telescopes are the most complex of all low vision aids and the most difficult to use correctly. Handheld varieties can and should be prescribed and taught by most low vision providers. Prescribing bioptics and telemicroscopes should only be attempted by experienced providers with a support staff of trained assistants including mobility instructors or occupational therapists. Such professionals are necessary to provide the follow-up training necessary for the successful use of these sophisticated devices.

Patients should be taught to use a telescope in several steps. First, the instructor should focus the telescope for infinity and teach the user the correct way to hold it (ie, with the ocular near the eye and the hand balanced against the face). Using two hands to hold the telescope provides more stability than one, and one arm or hand should be supported against a stationary object or the body. The patient should first view the distant object with the naked eye, then raise the telescope to view it more clearly. Always start with a well-lit object because the telescope blocks a great deal of light, and low contrast objects are thus very hard to see. Motion parallax will become evident very quickly, as well as the fact that objects appear to be much closer than they truly are. For these two reasons, instruct your patients not to attempt to walk while looking through the telescope. It should only be used while stationary.

After becoming proficient in spotting distant objects, your patient can be taught to change the focus for closer objects. Do this by picking out objects that are in the same line of view, both at least 15 feet away, and separated by at least 10 feet. Ask the patient to focus on the distant object, then view the nearer object, correcting the focus once it is in view. This should be practiced several times with different objects and varying distances. As practice progresses, the two chosen objects should be further apart. The most difficulty will be experienced when focusing from a very distant object to a very near one, or vice versa.

Once focusing is mastered, the patient can attempt scanning an area instead of only viewing a single object. This technique will be used when trying to take in a large field of view such as when watching sporting events or when trying to locate a person in a large room or field. The patient will learn to scan very slowly in order to overcome motion parallax and blurring. Instruct the patient to practice moving the telescope and his or her head as one unit. To practice the skill, several pictures or objects may be placed around a room, and the patient can be instructed to move his or her attention from one to the other. At first, the object should be placed at equal distances from the patient. As proficiency is gained some of the target objects should be closer than others, so the patient has to scan and focus at the same time.

The final skill to learn is tracking, or following a moving target. This skill will be necessary for watching an airplane take off or land, a person running a race, or any other moving object. The head and telescope are moved as one unit at the same speed as the moving target. Begin practice by following slow targets such as the instructor walking slowly. Gradually increase the speed of the moving object as the patient becomes more proficient.

Spotting, focusing, scanning, and tracking should each be taught separately and time allowed to practice between each of the tasks to develop proficiency. It may require several office visits before the individual becomes proficient with each of the skills and can use the telescope efficiently.

Addresses of Low Vision Aid Vendors

Rather than providing the address of every vendor of low vision aids, the following addresses should provide you with a wide variety of styles.

Eschenbach Optik of America
904 Ethan Allen Hwy
Ridgefield, CT 06877
800-487-5389
www.eschenbach.com

Independent Living Aids
PO Box 9022
Hicksville, NY 11802
800-537-2118
www.independentliving.com

Selsi
PO Box 10
Midland Park, NJ 07432
800-275-7357
www.selsioptics.com

For bioptic telescopes:
Designs for Vision
760 Koehler Ave
Ronkonkoma, NY 11779
800-727-6407
www.designsforvision.com

Helpful Web Sites

Vendors of Low Vision Magnifiers and Telescopes

- **Designs for Vision** (mostly bioptics and telescopic aids, good starter kits)
  www.designsforvision.com
- **Eschenbach Optik of America** (full-service company with hand magnifiers, stand magnifiers, telescopes, bioptics, and exam materials; they also offer training programs; good starter kits)
  www.eschenbach.com
- **Gulden Ophthalmics** (several magnifiers and writing aids)
  www.guldenindustries.com
- **Mons International** (vendor of aids from various companies, both optical and electronic)
  www.magnifiers.com/catalog
- **Selsi** (lower priced aids, telescopes, binocular scopes)
  www.selsioptics.com
- **S. Walters** (mostly telescopes, but some hand and stand magnifiers, good starter kits)
  www.walterslowvision.com

General Clearinghouses That Carry Many Brands of Aids

- **Independent Living Aids**
  www.independentliving.com

Information on Driving with Bioptics

- **Bioptic Driving Network**
  www.biopticdriving.org

Bibliography

Faye E, Hood C. *Low Vision.* Springfield, IL: Charles C. Thomas; 1975.

Fletcher D. *Low Vision Rehabilitation: Caring for the Whole Person.* San Francisco, CA: American Academy of Ophthalmology; 1999.

Fonda G. *Management of Low Vision.* New York, NY: Thieme-Stratton, Inc; 1981.

Freeman P, Jose R. *The Art and Practice of Low Vision.* 2nd ed. Burlington, MA: Butterworth-Heinemann; 1997.

Jose R. *Understanding Low Vision.* New York, NY: American Foundation for the Blind; 1983.

Peli E. *Driving With Confidence: A Practical Guide to Driving With Low Vision.* River Edge, NJ: World Scientific Publishing Co Pte Ltd; 2002.

Sloan L. *Recommended Aids for the Partially Sighted.* New York, NY: National Society for the Prevention of Blindness, Inc; 1971.

Wiener W, Vopata A. Suggested curriculum for distance training with optical aids. *The Journal of Visual Impairment and Blindness.* 1980;2:49-56.

Chapter 3

Non-Optical and Daily Living Aids

KEY POINTS

- Non-optical aids are available for reading, writing, medical use, and household use as well as for hobbies and games.

- Lighting is the most important non-optical aid.

- Many daily living aids are simply conveniences, but others are necessary for rehabilitation and a return to independent living.

Non-Optical Aids

A non-optical low vision aid is any device other than a magnifier that enables partially sighted or blind individuals to function more easily in their routine daily activities. Non-optical aids are numerous and include items as inexpensive as a simple sewing machine threader and as expensive and sophisticated as computerized voice-generated reading machines. This chapter will introduce non-electronic aids and appliances. Electronic devices are discussed in Chapter 4. Each non-optical aid has a specific use that enhances reading or tasks of daily living. A number of accessory devices provide increased contrast of reading materials. Other items incorporate larger print or are enlarged themselves, providing relative size magnification. Still others, such as audio or Braille versions of printed materials, provide assistance by avoiding visual limitations completely.

Many non-optical devices have nothing to do with printed material. They assist with daily activities such as eating, food preparation, and household organization. Frequently they are just adaptations of ordinary objects to make them safer or more manageable for people hindered by subnormal vision.

There are too many non-optical aids to mention individually, but an overview of the most common types follows.

Lighting

Light is the primary and most crucial non-optical device. Normally, visual acuity, color vision, and contrast sensitivity all decrease as available illumination diminishes. This decrease is exacerbated when a patient has a preexisting visual acuity loss.

Contrast sensitivity is one measure of the quality or efficiency of vision. It refers to the ability of the eye and brain to recognize images when the contrast between dark and light is diminished. Contrast sensitivity also decreases dramatically as acuity decreases, and low vision patients must find a way to improve contrast of written materials to see them more easily.

Most patients quickly realize that vision improves in sunlight and independently install higher watt lightbulbs in their lamps. This increased illumination is functional but not ideal. In order to be most effective, light must be strong enough to provide maximum contrast without bleaching out the print or causing glare. There are certain guidelines to guarantee that the light source a person uses will give the best illumination. Boyce and Sanford recommend that the specifics to look for are lamps that have good color rendering properties and very little light output below 450 nanometers (nm). The user should have no view of the light source itself either directly or by reflection. The shade should be highly reflective to provide uniform illumination and soften shadows.[1]

Some lights are better than others at reproducing true colors. This color rendering ability is measured by the color rendering index (CRI). The CRI number of a particular light source determines what percent of the actual color of an object is reproduced accurately under a particular lighting situation. A CRI of 100 is optimum. Generally, fluorescent bulbs have a CRI between approximately 55 and 75. Incandescent bulbs of 75 watts have a CRI of 100.

All light contains colors as determined by the wavelengths of particular rays. The light output of every lamp has various levels of these differing wavelengths of light, therefore allowing the resolution of some colors better than others. These wavelengths are measured in nanometers, or nm. (A nanometer is one billionth of a meter.) The human eye can only discern colors of the rainbow, which contain light rays between 400 and 700 nm. This is referred to as the visible light spectrum. The lower end of our visible light spectrum is the violet range, which is just above the

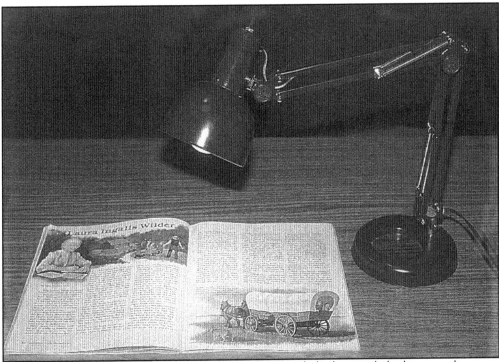

Figure 3-1. A traditional form of task lighting with a metal shade. Metal shades are only recommended when the reader does not need to be in close proximity to the lamp, since the shade can become quite hot.

wavelengths of ultraviolet (UV) light. Since UVA and UVB rays have been found to be damaging to the retina, it is best for the majority of rays from any light sources to be well away from the UV range (100 to 400 nm).

Although everyone benefits from optimum lighting, when comparing various ocular diagnoses patients with ARMD receive the greatest increase in acuity under improved light conditions.[1] For these patients, increased illumination will improve vision for reading as well as for general moving about the home. One log unit of increase in illumination increases contrast sensitivity by 1.5 dB and increases visual acuity by 0.13 logMAR units.[2] This represents the ability to see letters that are approximately 25% smaller than can be easily read without proper illumination, which for many patients is a significant improvement. The additional advantage of good light is that as it increases acuity and contrast sensitivity it allows for a lower power magnifier to be used thus allowing for increased reading distance and a wider field of view.

For most ARMD patients, a 60-watt incandescent bulb is ideal for optimum contrast. Lower powers do not provide enough light and higher powers cause glare. The bulb is most efficient when used in a reflective shade (generally cone shaped) that directs 100% of the available light onto the page (Figure 3-1).

No matter what type of reading lamp is chosen, there must be some flexibility in the stand or arm of the lamp for optimum positioning. Any gooseneck or movable arm type of lamp (usually referred to as a task light) will do as long as it allows the light to be shone directly onto the page of print. Unless a magnifier causes the need for more precise positioning, light at a 45-degree angle from the print and placed on the same side as the preferred eye is recommended for normal use. When using a magnifier, the more flexible the arm of the lamp the better, as sometimes the

Figure 3-2. An Ott-Lite™ provides more natural "full-spectrum" light from a bulb that generates very little heat, glare, or shadow.

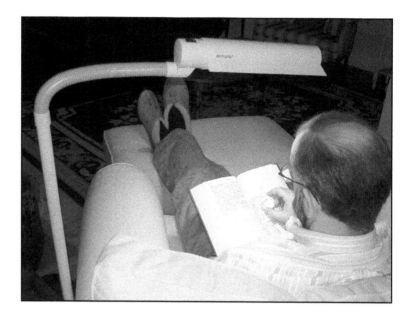

Figure 3-3. Ott-Lites come in many fashionable styles as well as the utilitarian versions, providing improved illumination in the entire home, not just at the reading desk. (Photo courtesy of Ott-Lite Technology, Tampa, FL.)

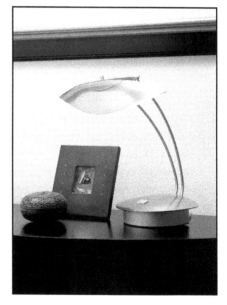

shade must be brought very close to the reading material and angled precisely to eliminate any shadows caused by the patient's arm or by the housing of a magnifier.

These lamps are available widely in office supply stores. The least expensive varieties are fine for most uses, but higher priced varieties have the advantage of an insulated shade. This insulated shade is better for patients who view objects very close to their face and stay in close proximity to the lamp for a long time. The insulation keeps the shade cooler and helps prevent burns.

Another type of lamp preferred by patients for reading and household use is the Ott-Lite™ (Ott-Lite Technology, Tampa, FL). These are special fluorescent lamps designed to mimic the full spectrum of daylight illumination indoors, thereby enhancing color vision and contrast sensitivity (Figures 3-2 and 3-3). They are used for crafting and other hobbies that require excellent vision and accurate color matching because they have an excellent CRI of 85. Because Ott-Lites and other full-spectrum bulbs are fluorescent, they generate less heat and the bulbs last longer than incandescent bulbs. They also provide light using lower watt bulbs (about 13 to 25 watts) and so create fewer shadows and less glare.

There has been some criticism of these lights because the way they provide more optimum color rendering is to include more of the violet wavelengths of light. Incandescent bulbs are in the 550 to 700 nm range which is the more yellow-red portion and explains the yellow cast to the light they provide. Full-spectrum fluorescent bulbs also include rays in the 400 to 470 nm range. The effect of the brighter light they provide is due in some part to the enhancement of white objects due to the "UV glow" they provide rather than to actually increasing the brightness of the light. There is some concern raised on low vision patient blogs and web sites that since they emit more light near the UV part of the spectrum that they can be damaging to the eyes. However, compared to the level of UV rays in the sunlight the level in Ott-Lites is extremely minimal. The Ott-Lite only emits 0.2 microwatts of power in the UV spectrum. Also, the violet wavelengths that they incorporate are most highly concentrated in the 450 nm range, which has been shown to be acceptable for low vision use. The advantages of these lights are the enhanced color rendering, less heat generated by the bulb, less glare and shadows, a long-lasting bulb, and flexible positioning. The disadvantages are that they emit some rays near the UV spectrum and carry a higher cost than normal incandescent bulbs. Although the evaluation of the advantages vs disadvantages should be considered individually, full-spectrum lights are frequently recommended for low vision patients. No matter what type of bulb you use, elderly patients need to be reassured that a close light source will not harm their eyes. Many of them were raised believing that too much light or too much reading can be the cause of blindness.

Distributors of reading lamps for low vision:
Lighting Specialties
735 Hastings Lane
Buffalo Grove, IL 60089
800-214-4522
www.lightspc.com

Ott-Lites are available through retailers, but the company address is:
Ott-Lite Technology
1214 W Cass St
Tampa, FL 33606
800-842-8848
www.ottlite.com

Not all patients benefit from a direct light source. It is important to experiment with illumination positions and styles for each individual to determine what is optimal for each patient. Although persons with macular degeneration benefit greatly from increasing illumination, cataract and post-laser diabetic retinopathy patients often experience *decreased* acuity as the light intensifies due to scatter and glare. Patients with ocular albinism and aniridia are very light sensitive and prefer conditions with lower illumination. Task lighting is still the best choice, but will be more useful if moved further from the page or when using a lower power bulb to decrease the light level. These patients also benefit from other non-optical aids such as sunglasses and light-absorbing filters.

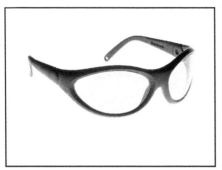

Figure 3-4. NoIR™ provides many styles of sunglasses with varying levels of light absorption. (Photo courtesy of NoIR Medical Technologies, South Lyon, MI.)

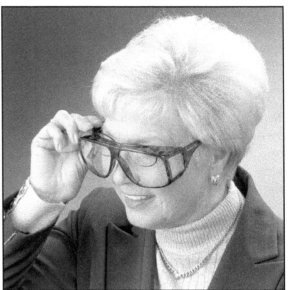

Figure 3-5. Sunglasses with yellow lenses can be used to increase the contrast of reading material. (Photo courtesy of Eschenbach Optik of America, Ridgefield, CT.)

Filters and Sun Protection

Special sunglasses that wrap around the patient's face and filter light from all angles are popular with low vision patients (Figures 3-4 and 3-5). SolarShields® (Dioptics, San Luis Obispo, CA) and NoIR™ (NoIR Medical Technologies, South Lyon, MI) sunglasses are the best known varieties. Their design prevents glare in most light situations. Levels of protection vary from light tints with only UV protection to the most dense tints that allow transmission of only 2% of available light. Green or brown tints are good for decreasing light levels and to eliminate glare. Yellow enhances contrast and is useful for improving the readability of printed material, particularly blue ink. School children may use them to improve contrast of photocopied sheets at school. A piece of letter-sized yellow acetate film placed on photocopied paper provides the same service if a child does not want to wear unusual sunglasses. Optical shops can tint the patient's standard prescription lenses for increased contrast or light protection as well.

Absorptive filter lenses are recommended particularly for patients with albinism, retinitis pigmentosa, and glaucoma. Patients who have undergone cataract extraction or retinal laser treatment also benefit from their use. Some patients prefer light tints for indoors and darker tints for outdoors. Patients with poor contrast resolution as a result of ischemic optic neuropathy or glaucoma benefit from yellow-tinted glasses. Visors or hats with wide brims also protect the eyes from the brightness of the sun and can increase visual efficiency outdoors.

Yellow filters can be ordered from non-optical aids suppliers such as Independent Living Aids (Hicksville, NY) or LS&S (Northbrook, IL). Absorptive sunglasses may be ordered from the following companies by mail or online:

Dioptics
125 Venture Dr
San Luis Obispo, CA 93401
805-781-3300
www.dioptics.com

NoIR Medical Technologies
PO Box 159
South Lyon, MI 48178
800-521-9746
www.noir-medical.com

Patients with peripheral retinal degenerations may become debilitated in low light situations and become essentially "night blind." Night vision spotting scopes (originally designed for the military and regularly used by hunters) detect infrared and other ambient light and electronically make a scene appear bright even in very low light conditions. These are available as small hand-held scopes or scopes worn on the head to help people see at night or when entering a darkened room.

To find further information on night vision scopes, or for ordering, contact:
American Technologies Network
20 S Linden Ave, Suite 1B
South San Francisco, CA 94080
800-910-2862
www.atncorp.com

What the Patient Needs to Know

- Brighter lightbulbs are not the only answer to help you read better. Sometimes a lower watt bulb is better. In either case, the illumination should shine directly on the subject matter.

- Light can be placed in any location that provides optimal contrast of the print. It is not necessarily best if it comes over your shoulder from behind.

- Bright light on a page of print will not harm your eyes.

- If glare is a problem for you, it is okay to move your reading light further away or wear sunglasses indoors.

Reading and Writing Aids

"Large print" is a term that applies to any size print larger than the standard. In books, magazines, and newspapers large print generally refers to 16- to 18-point type, which is $2\times$ magnification, or twice the size of "regular" print (Figure 3-6). The United States Postal Service uses 18-point type as their official minimum size for large print that can be mailed without postage as "free matter for the blind."

Figure 3-6. Large print as it relates to X notation and font size.

Large Print	
Magnification	Correlated Font Size
1X	10 pt
2X	16 pt
3X	26 pt
4X	36 pt
5X	44 pt
11X	92 pt

Large-print books, magazines, and newspapers are widely available. They can eliminate the need for optical devices for patients with moderately low vision and may be the only reading material possible for those with severe vision loss who use strong magnifiers. Local libraries carry many bestsellers and popular titles in large print. Several agencies, such as the National Library Service for the Blind and Physically Handicapped and the National Association for Visually Handicapped (address on page 47), have large-print lending libraries that can be accessed through the mail. Most reference books such as dictionaries and atlases are commercially available in large-print editions as well. In collaboration with the American Foundation for the Blind, *The New York Times* is published in a condensed large-print edition called *The New York Times Large Type Weekly*. Magazines available in large-print include *Reader's Digest* (Figure 3-7), *Reader's Digest Select Editions* (which provides two bestselling books every other month), and *Guideposts* inspirational magazine. The following resources are good places to start:

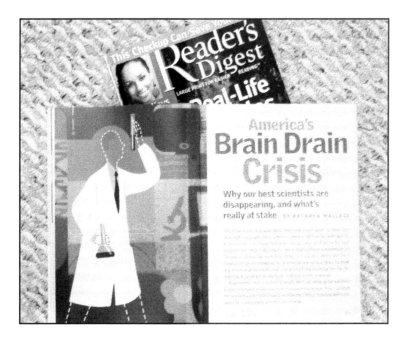

Figure 3-7. *Reader's Digest Large Print for Easier Reading Edition*™ is one of many magazines available in large type.

National Library Service for the Blind and Physically Handicapped
The Library of Congress
888-657-7323
www.loc.gov/nls

(The street address in Washington, DC does not receive mail—call or use the web site to find a branch near you, or contact your local librarian for details.)

The New York Times Large Type Weekly
The New York Times Co
PO Box 9564
Uniondale, NY 11555
800–631-2580
www.nytimes.com/ref/membercenter/help

Reader's Digest Large Print for Easier Reading Edition (monthly)
PO Box 8177
Red Oak, IA 51591
800-807-2780
www.rd.com

Most school textbooks are available in, or can be converted to, large print or Braille. Contact:

American Printing House for the Blind
PO Box 6085
Louisville, KY 40206
800-223-1839
www.aph.org

Figure 3-8. Using a check writing guide and a 20/20 pen™ makes it easier to maintain independence in personal finances and record keeping.

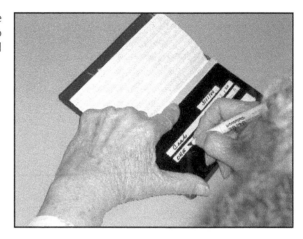

Figure 3-9. Reading stands come in many varieties. They help position reading material for use with a magnifier while maintaining a comfortable body position. (Photo courtesy of Eschenbach Optik of America, Ridgefield, CT.)

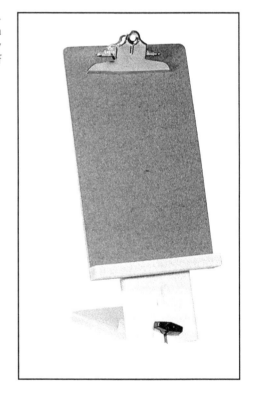

Line isolators (typoscopes) are heavy plastic or metal strips with rectangular sections cut out which isolate one or two lines of print on a page. These eliminate all distracting background print when reading or writing. They are commercially available or may be homemade of laminated black construction paper or posterboard. Some are pocket size with an opening only big enough for a signature and allow patients to "sign on the dotted line" without having to see the dotted line. Some are cut as stencils appropriate for addressing envelopes or writing checks (Figure 3-8).

Reading stands sit on a table or desk and hold reading material at a proper height and angle. They promote a more comfortable posture for the very close reading distances necessary when using low vision aids. They also support the book, freeing one hand for reading with a magnifier (Figure 3-9). A reading lamp can be situated next to a reading stand so the optimum light is always available where it is needed. Many patients find this system invaluable in reducing stress

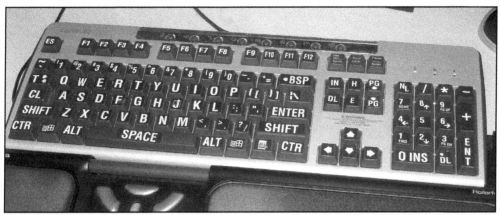

Figure 3-10. Special stickers can be applied to convert a normal keyboard to large print. These stickers come in white on black or black on yellow for high contrast. They are preprinted and precut to fit the keys of any standard keyboard.

and effort when reading with optical low vision aids. There are many styles of reading stands commercially available, or patients can build their own if they prefer a simpler design.

Black felt-tip markers draw lines that are read more easily than those from pens and pencils. Low vision patients should keep a supply on hand and instruct their friends and family members to use them in correspondence. Low vision supply vendors also sell bold-lined writing paper, which is lined like notebook paper, but with bold black lines. School children find this very helpful when learning to write, as the lines on standard writing tablets have very low contrast and are extremely difficult to see.

Medical Devices

Many medical devices have been adapted to enable people with low vision to remain involved in their own home care, particularly persons with diabetes. Some of the adapted devices available include:

- Syringes with magnifiers attached
- Syringes with large-print characters
- Talking blood glucose monitors
- Adapters for medicine vials to center the needle correctly
- Talking blood pressure cuffs
- Talking thermometers
- Large-print, Braille, and talking pill boxes
- Talking Rx medicine bottle readers that read name and dosage

Homecare and Cooking

Non-optical aids for the home include items to help with keeping time, doing personal business tasks, cooking, cleaning, and grooming. Some of the many daily living aids that are available include:

- Large-print, Braille, and talking clocks and watches
- Large-print stickers for computer keyboards (Figure 3-10)

Figure 3-11. Large print playing cards come in many varieties. These are Marinoff Low Vision Playing Cards™. They include large print in two different sizes and high contrast (because of the black outlines around the numbers).

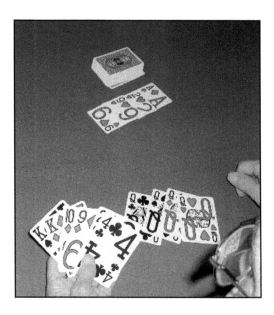

- Talking alarm clocks
- Talking calculators
- Telephones with large-print buttons
- Large-print address books
- Rulers with bold large-print numbers
- Bump-ons, which are small rubber adhesive dots for labeling dials and knobs
- Flame tamers for the stove to prevent burning
- Talking egg timers, microwaves, and ovens
- Liquid level indicators to prevent overfilling of cups and glasses
- Bread knives with attached guides to measure the slices and protect fingers
- Wallet organizers to separate bills of different denominations

Hobbies and Games

There are also many adapted games, sewing supplies, tools, and other recreational materials including:

- Automatic needle threaders and spread-eye needles
- Magnifiers that attach to sewing machines for assistance with threading
- Tape measures with tactile markings—both for sewing and for woodwork
- Measuring levels with electronic audio signals when they are level
- Talking stud finders
- Talking tire gauges
- Large-print playing cards (Figure 3-11)
- Balls with audible beeps for easy localization (available for most sports)
- Other beeping accessories for sports including baseball bases
- Backgammon and other games in large-print and Braille versions (Figure 3-12)
- Many talking electronic and computer games

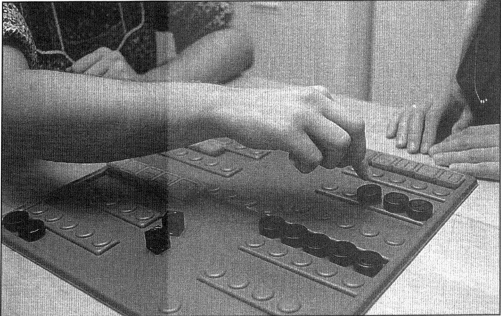

Figure 3-12. A tactile Backgammon® game can be enjoyed by sighted, partially sighted, or blind players.

Braille

Usually low vision providers think in terms of providing larger print or higher power magnifiers to patients. It is easy to forget that there is a time when Braille becomes the best choice, or even an alternate one for written communication. The Braille "alphabet" was devised by Louis Braille, a blind musician and gifted student in France in the mid-19th century. His inspiration came from a method of night communication for Louis XVIII's Army, which Braille transformed as a code of writing for blind students.[3] The dotted "code" spread quickly for use as a means of written communication by blind people across the world. The six dots in a Braille cell (two across, three down) are arranged in various combinations, each of which stands for a letter, number, or group of letters (such as "ing" or "tion"). Books and magazines are available in Braille for adults and children, and unavailable titles and texts can be converted to Braille. Conversion is time-consuming, so orders for specific school texts must be submitted far in advance of when classes begin. Teachers and parents need to plan ahead. Contact the American Printing House for the Blind (address on page 41) or:

National Braille Press
88 St Stephen St
Boston, MA 02115
888-965-8965
www.nbp.org

Figure 3-13. The Perkins Brailler is a classic machine that is used like a type-writer but embosses paper with Braille cells.

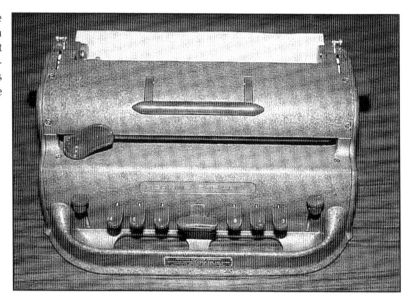

An individual can write using Braille symbols with a rather cumbersome apparatus called a Braille Writer (or Perkins Brailler), which looks and functions like a manual typewriter (Figure 3-13). For more portable writing, notes can be taken with the use of a small stencil and punch, called a "slate and stylus." With a Braille slate and stylus, metal Braille "stickers" can be individually punched and applied to CDs, games, and appliances as labels so blind individuals can locate their belongings. In addition, the "on/off" and "volume" switches can be labeled on an MP3 or CD player for easier location if they are not already differentiated by the manufacturer with raised markings. Most of us have seen these stickers labeling the floor numbers near elevator buttons in public buildings.

Some patients find it difficult to differentiate the various Braille symbols. The dots are close together and are raised only slightly off the smooth paper. The fingers of some adult patients are too large to locate the small dots accurately. Diabetics have decreased sensation to their extremities and have difficulty detecting the bumps. Some cannot sense the raised dots at all. Other patients simply cannot learn the new "language." Braille is not for everyone, but should not be forgotten as a possible and excellent alternative for some patients.

Non-optical aids that do not have specific addresses listed in this chapter can be ordered by catalogue from distributors who carry a large variety of aids. Order your free catalogues from the following:

Independent Living Aids
PO Box 9022
Hicksville, NY 11802
800-537-2118
www.independentliving.com

LS&S
PO Box 673
Northbrook, IL 60065
800-468-4789
www.lssproducts.com

Maxi-Aids
42 Executive Blvd
Farmingdale, NY 11735
800-522-6294
www.maxiaids.com

National Association for Visually Handicapped
22 W 21st St, 6th Floor
New York, NY 10010
212-255-2804
        or
507 Polk St, Suite 420
San Francisco, CA 94102
415-775-6284
www.navh.org

Helpful Web Sites

Vendors of Daily Living Aids

- **Active and Able** (adaptive aids for many disabilities)
  www.activeandable.com/catalog
- **American Printing House for the Blind** (mainly educational materials)
  www.aph.org
- **Independent Living Aids** (a huge catalogue of adaptive devices and optical aids)
  www.independentliving.com
- **The Low Vision Store** (aids and appliances for sale online to the consumer)
  www.thelowvisionstore.com
- **Maxi-Aids** (clearinghouse of many daily living aids by catalogue and online)
  www.maxiaids.com/store
- **Sight Connection** (large supply of non-optical and assistive devices)
  www.sightconnection.com

Lighting Needs

- **Ott-Lite Technology** (informational, refers you to vendors)
  www.ottlite.com
- **Sun and light filters**
  www.noir-medical.com (NoIR sunglasses)
  www.dioptics.com/brands_solarshield.html (SolarShields)
- **Task lighting** (clearinghouse for many brands of lights)
  www.lightspc.com

Large-Print Materials

- **Braille Works** (prints books in large print or Braille)
  http://brailleworks.com
- **Harvard Ranch Publishing** (religious and devotional books in large print)
  www.harvardranch.com
- **Huge Print Press** (prints any book in any size font)
  www.hugeprint.com
- **Jewish Braille Institute** (creates books, magazines, cultural programs in large print or Braille or in audio in seven languages)
  www.jewishbraille.org
- **Talking Book Productions** (creates professionally recorded versions of any text)
  www.talkingbookproductions.com

References

1. Boyce P, Sanford L. *Lighting to Enhance Visual Capabilities. The Lighthouse Handbook on Vision Impairment and Vision Rehabilitation.* Vol I. New York, NY: Oxford University Press; 2000:617-636.

2. Haymes S, Lee J. Effects of task lighting on visual function in age-related macular degeneration. *Ophthalmic Physiol Opt.* 2006;26:169-179.

3. Wallechinsky D, Wallace I. *The People's Almanac.* Garden City, NY: Doubleday and Co; 1975:520-521.

Bibliography

Eperjesi F, Fowler C, Evans B. Do tinted lenses or filters improve visual performance in low vision? A review of the literature. *Ophthalmic Physiol Opt.* 2002;22:68-77.

International Commission on Illumination (Commission Internationale de L'Elairage). *Technical Report: Low Vision, Lighting Needs for the Partially Sighted.* CIE publication 123-1997.

Leat S, Woo G. The validity of current clinical tests of contrast sensitivity and their ability to predict reading speed in low vision. *Eye.* 1997;11:893-899.

McGillivray R. Comprehensive computer access evaluation for persons with low vision. *Aids and Appliances Review.* 1994;15:2-8.

Stetten D. Sounding board: coping with blindness. *N Engl J Med.* 1981;305:458-460.

Chapter 4

Electronic and Computer-Assisted Low Vision Aids

KEY POINTS

- Electronic assistive devices for the low vision/blind patient include electronic magnification systems, computer programs, synthesized speech, speech compression, and other electronic daily living aids.

- Advances in technology are creating opportunities in communication and Internet support for people with visual disabilities.

- Accessibility options are a common part of computer operating systems.

- Most low vision patients should be considered as candidates for electronic aids, regardless of their age or background.

Introduction

The current era of sophisticated electronics has affected the quality of life of low vision patients by opening up a world of communication they were unable to experience before. When electronic devices are designed specifically for the handicapped, they are referred to as *assistive* or *adaptive technology*. Assistive devices for people with visual handicaps make it possible to enlarge the print of any written material or to turn written text into synthesized speech (eg, read aloud by a computer). Some machines also provide the reverse ability, transferring spoken words into written form via a computer interface. Using electronics, computer programs can be altered so the visually impaired can use the Internet. Some of these machines and appliances are so sophisticated that they require trained instructors to work with the patients. Others are so user-friendly that any low vision provider can offer them to patients and expect good results.

Assistive technology devices for the visually impaired fall into four basic categories:
1. Computer programs or electronic vision enhancement systems such as CCTVs or other devices that electronically enlarge print
2. Optical character recognition (OCR) with which written text can be scanned and recognized by a computer
3. Speech synthesizers which transfer written text into the spoken word
4. Digital recording which manipulates the spoken word so that it can be interfaced with computer programs or easily controlled for speed and frequency

Like all electronic devices, those for use by visually impaired people continue to improve and become more compact every year. Because of decreasing cost and better portability of these devices, as well as the ability to vary magnification levels from 3× to as high as 70×, they are becoming more common and desired by a large segment of the low vision population. It has also been shown that reading speed and duration is better with electronic magnifiers than with traditional optical aids.[1] Because of this, they may be preferred for the patient with extensive reading needs vs optical aids that are better designed for short-term use. Since electronic devices become obsolete fairly quickly, it is strongly recommended that the reader investigate any electronic aids listed in this book by contacting the manufacturer before prescribing them or suggesting their use to low vision patients. Verify that the device still exists and also explore whether an improved version is available.

For a complete and up-to-date listing of electronic assistive devices, log on to the American Foundation for the Blind (AFB) web site and access their technology center.

Electronic Magnification Systems

Desktop Closed Circuit Televisions

The most common electronic low vision aid, and the one that has been in use for the longest time, is the CCTV. The traditional CCTV consists of a video monitor with a small video camera attached beneath it or installed internally. Written material is placed on a movable x,y platform under the camera, where it is instantly filmed and transmitted onto the monitor in large print (Figure 4-1). The print size is variable and the limit of enlargement is specific to each machine. Some CCTVs only enlarge type to 11× while others can provide up to 70× magnification. As the magnification becomes larger the field of view becomes smaller, so at the higher magnification

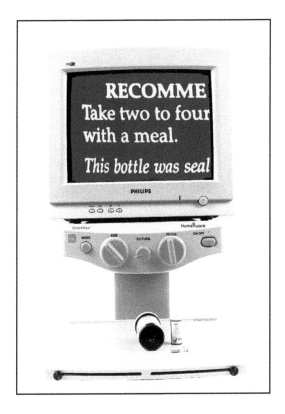

Figure 4-1. The Smartview 3000™ desktop model CCTV showing a reverse polarity screen and an x,y table. (Photo courtesy of HumanWare, Concord, CA.)

levels a larger monitor will provide the ability to visualize more letters at a time, maintaining a wide field of view.

The hard copy must be moved below the camera while reading, which is sometimes difficult for users to master. Sometimes tracking the page back and forth causes smearing or jerking of the print. A slower tracking speed is helpful to eliminate this problem, and models are continually redesigned to minimize it as well. The other difficulty that people encounter at first is controlling the x,y table. When the surface can move forward, backward, left, and right all at once it tends to move around a little bit uncontrollably until the user has had adequate training and practice.

There are many advantages of CCTVs. They enable patients to read materials that are not otherwise available in large print. The user is free to adopt a preferred head position for best vision. The machines are adapted for writing as well as reading. Such aids are also excellent for viewing illustrations, photographs, or collectibles such as coins and stamps.

CCTV features vary, but some are fairly standard. Many models offer a choice of screen displays. The traditional screen is a white background with black print. Reverse polarity displays provide a black background with white print for better contrast and glare control. Full-color screens are available in most models for viewing photographs and color documents. Many CCTVs allow users to choose a background color that is most compatible with their individual vision needs. For example, a patient might choose a yellow background to increase contrast or a gray background to diminish it. A shadow masking feature allows the screen to be narrowed or darkened so only one line of print is illuminated. Line markers allow the reader to electronically underline print on the monitor (Figure 4-2). These features can be useful to track pertinent information or simply to maintain one's place on the page. One disadvantage is that the line marker or masking window stays in a constant position and the user must move the printed material while

Figure 4-2. Aladdin Pro™ CCTV monitor showing a line marker in use.

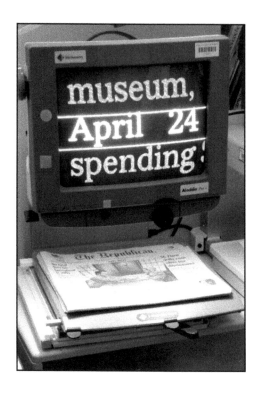

trying to keep the important information within the limits of the marker. This is not very easy with a movable x,y platform.

The price of standard CCTVs is between $1,500 and $3,000 with higher prices as more options are added.

Portable Systems

Newer versions of CCTVs are smaller than the standard tabletop models. They provide versatility and portability that is more useful for many people. Some have smaller camera stands and a separate monitor. Since these systems are so easy to take along and adaptable, they are generally sold without a monitor. They are equipped with only a camera stand, which is then attached to any television or computer monitor. Systems such as Clarity's PCMate™ and Carrymate™ (Minden, NV) can be attached to any computer and used for distance viewing (Figure 4-3). When attached to a laptop or notebook computer, they can be used in a boardroom or classroom to view chalkboards, projector screens, and speakers through the computer monitor, eliminating the need for wearing a telescopic correction. They can also be aimed at near to help with writing or with reading text. The price of these portable CCTVs is generally in the same range as the desktop models.

There are several other types of versatile electronic readers. The Max Digital Magnifier™ (Enhanced Vision, Huntington Beach, CA) is a small handheld digital reader. The hand unit is run over the printed material like an optical mouse. This scans the print which can then be seen on a viewing screen. The Max can be attached to any monitor or television and comes in color or black and white versions (Figure 4-4). It provides magnification of 16× to 28×. The MaxPort version attaches to a pair of electronic viewing spectacles which function as a head-born monitor, and thus can be taken anywhere. The Max Panel edition comes with its own LCD screen, but must

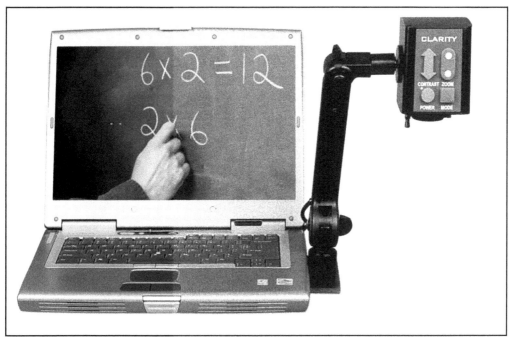

Figure 4-3. Clarity PCMate™ attached to a laptop for classroom use. (Photo courtesy of Clarity, Minden, NV.)

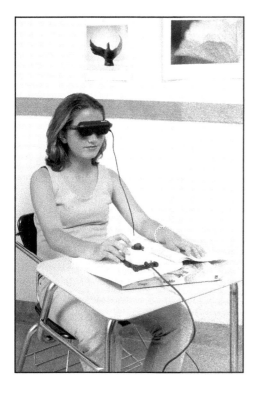

Figure 4-4. The Max™ can be used at work or school. With the viewing spectacles, no monitor is necessary. (Photo courtesy of Enhanced Vision, Huntington Beach, CA.)

Figure 4-5. JORDY™ in use for distance viewing.

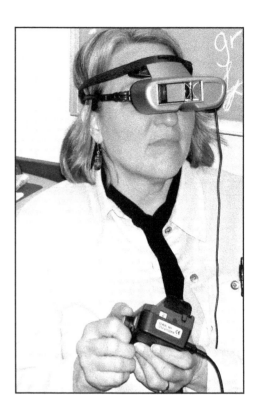

be used on a tabletop. The Max Reader (without attachments) is relatively inexpensive (around $400 to $500), easily transported, and handy for reading small items like recipe cards and mail. It can also read from curved surfaces as well as flat, and so can be used for tasks such as reading the labels on cans or prescription bottles.

The Flipper™ (Enhanced Vision) is a portable and lightweight CCTV that must be attached to a monitor or to optional viewing spectacles. It can be used for distance viewing as well as near reading. The video camera portion is mounted on a flexible hinge that is movable across 225 degrees of rotation. This allows versatile use since most any location in a room can be viewed just by moving the video head. It is designed for near tasks, but can also be used to view in the distance by flipping up the head to point at a distant object. The machine is able to provide up to 50× magnification at near and 24× at distance.

Another device, the JORDY™ system (Enhanced Vision) is designed specifically to be worn as a headset (Figure 4-5). It is worn over prescription lenses and can focus near or far, providing up to 30× magnification at near and in the distance. The eyepieces have viewing screens (instead of lenses) which are attached to a small camera on the front of the system. The material being viewed is seen inside the eyepieces much like a virtual reality headset, allowing a 44-degree field of view. Alternately, the headset can be attached to a computer monitor and the image can be viewed on the screen for up to 50× magnification. The JORDY is controlled by a small battery pack which is worn on the belt or in a pocket. It also comes with a tabletop docking unit so the headset can be installed over an x,y table to be used more like a traditional CCTV. A disadvantage to the JORDY is that the headset, although it only weighs 8 ounces, feels heavy and uncomfortable over time. It also blocks peripheral vision and the viewer can only see what is within the headset while it is in use. The flexibility of being able to view distance or near is a plus. The JORDY system is priced in the $3,000 range.

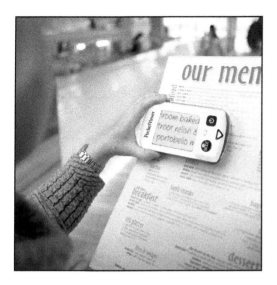

Figure 4-6. The PocketViewer™ by Human-Ware. (Photo courtesy of Eschenbach Optik of America, Ridgefield, CT.)

Handheld electronic magnifiers are extremely portable. These are small battery-operated video magnifiers that look something like a handheld video game. They can be held over any object or any print and magnify it on the attached screen. Magnification levels vary from 4× up to 26×. Some of these systems are useful not only for reading, but also for writing as when filling out forms or writing checks. The Pico™ from Telesensory (Malaysia) has a setting that allows a pen and paper to be positioned beneath it for easy viewing. Batteries provide over an hour of continuous use between charges, so the Pico, with its autofocus feature, is good for shopping or traveling. Optelec (Vista, CA) makes an analogous portable magnifier called the Traveller™ which is designed for reading with the addition of a writing feature.

Telesensory's Olympia™ portable magnifier is similar to the Pico but slightly larger and heavier (2.5 lbs). It provides up to 26× magnification and has a 7-inch diagonal screen. It can be attached to a video monitor as well for even larger magnification. The Pocketmate™ by Clarity and PocketViewer™ (Figure 4-6) by HumanWare (Concord, CA) are also comparable to the Pico. They are small handheld battery-operated video magnifiers with a 4-inch fixed focus LCD screen and a small carrying case.

Computer Programs and Synthesized Speech

Computer and Internet access can be frustrating and difficult for low vision patients because many of the characters and icons are too small to be easily seen. Windows™ (Microsoft Corp, Redmond, WA) and Apple™ (Cupertino, CA) operating systems both provide accessibility options that allow the user to enlarge the size of print on the screen as well as icons and other features so they can be more successfully navigated by the low vision user (Figure 4-7). (For information on how to access this option go to www.microsoft.com/enable or www.apple.com.) Using a larger monitor is also helpful to expand what is seen on the screen. However, these enlargement and accessibility functions have limitations and are not satisfactory for all users, particularly those with more severe vision loss.

An alternative to the standard accessibility options provided with operating systems is to install one of the specialized magnification software packages designed specifically for low vision use. When these programs are installed into a personal computer, they allow the user to see

Figure 4-7. A computer monitor showing enlarged screen displays available through the standard accessibility options in Windows™.

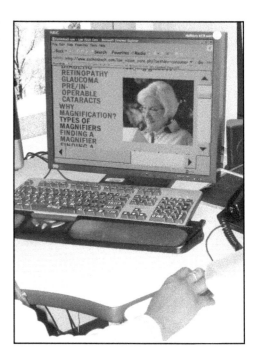

other software programs and web sites in larger print. These magnifiers automatically provide up to 32× magnification of all print, spreadsheets, and graphics on the Internet and in all software applications. The advantage to using this type of program over simply using a larger font size is that the toolbar is also shown in larger sizes, as is the mouse pointer and all icons. In addition, functions are included that are very helpful in navigating around a document while only viewing an enlarged portion of it. The print size can be changed from 2× to 16× at the touch of a key. These programs can be used with current word processing programs, accounting programs, the Internet, and email.

Many screen magnification programs also include optical character recognition (OCR) features and/or a speech synthesizer. OCR enables a machine to scan and translate the printed word. Synthesized speech then says words aloud as they appear on the screen. The combination of OCR and synthesized speech is referred to as a text-to-speech program. The synthesized voices are artificial, but are easy to understand. Pronunciation is usually accurate, although the computer might misinterpret some words, especially when they are used out of context or are abbreviations (eg, saying "corn" instead of "com" when reading web sites with a dot-com ending), but primarily the translation and pronunciation are both reliable. Some synthesizers are better than others and sound more like natural voices. Speech-adapted computer programs are excellent for patients with severe disabilities. They are also good for users with better vision but for whom computer-induced eye fatigue is a problem or who have a physical inability to sit for long periods of time in front of a computer monitor.

ZoomText 9.0™ from Ai Squared (Manchester Center, VT) is a popular and user-friendly software package for use with Windows™ that provides magnification up to 36×. It includes speech synthesizers in 15 languages. Other similar programs from Freedom Scientific (St Petersburg, FL) are OpenBook™ which provides large-print and synthesized speech, JAWS™ for Windows which provides a speech synthesizer and Braille displays, and MAGic 9.5™ which offers magnification with or without the speech component. The Supernova™, Lunar™, and Lunar

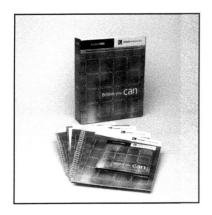

Figure 4-8. Kurzweil 1000™ program. (Photo courtesy of Kurzweil Educational Systems, Bedford, MA.)

Plus™ screen magnifiers from Optelec work with Windows Platforms™ for PC computers. The InLarge™ program from ALVA Access Group (Optelec) is designed to be used with MacIntosh™ systems.

Kurzweil Education Systems (Bedford, MA) offers two programs for educational use. The Kurzweil 1000™ is a program that contains a text-to-speech feature as well as enlarged print and highlighting capabilities (Figures 4-8 and 4-9). It also includes editing tools and provides other study skills such as note taking, summarizing, and outlining. The program can access online devices such as encyclopedias, talking newspapers, and other study aids. The information can then be downloaded into an MP3 or Daisy player for future use. (See page 59 for more information about Daisy players.) It can also print in embossed Braille. The Kurzweil 3000™ is a similar program for students with other types of learning or reading disabilities. It is designed for use with Windows or MacIntosh and includes features such as highlighting, access to word meanings, and writing tools.

AT&T™ sponsors a text-to-speech program called NaturalReader™ (NaturalSoft Ltd, Vancouver, BC, Canada) in which a preferred synthesized voice can be chosen from a selection of males and females, both American and British. They also have French, Spanish, and German versions, and the voices can be adjusted for speed and quality. Also, the recordings can be downloaded to an MP3 player for future listening. One advantage of the NaturalReader is that a simplified version can be downloaded for free from the company's web site (see end of chapter).

Apple™ markets an operating system for MacIntosh computers called Mac OS X™ which provides many accessibility options all in one package including reverse polarity, grayscale, and enhanced contrast screen displays. Print can be magnified up to 20× with a feature that allows for zooming in and out of selected sections of the screen. The VoiceOver™ component of Mac OS X provides a text-to-speech synthesizer, an onscreen scientific calculator, and a built-in dictionary and thesaurus. A translation feature can be activated while writing or editing a document so the author can hear what is currently being written or edited. The program also allows for multiple users to choose their own individual settings which will be saved and will automatically reformat to the individual preferences when that person logs on to the computer. Mac OS X is available directly through the Apple web site or by phone.

Figure 4-9. Example of on-screen outlining features from the Kurzweil 1000™ program. (Photo courtesy of Kurzweil Educational Systems, Bedford, MA.)

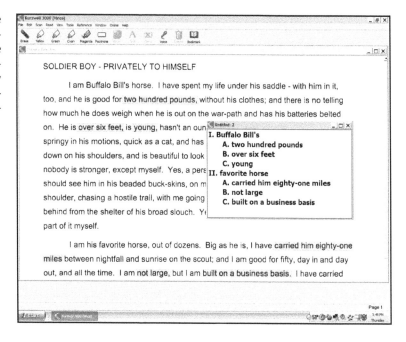

The Microsoft XP operating system provides accessibility for the visually impaired that allows control of the size of the scrollbars, desktop icons, and window borders. It also allows for changes in contrast and polarity as well as the size, color, and blink rate of the mouse cursor. In the Microsoft Vista system, the terminology is changed from accessibility options to the "Ease of Access Center." It includes improvements in the method of magnification as well as speech recognition features and other improved accessibility options.

Blind users may also benefit from two other assistive devices, the Braille display and voice-activated controls. When attached to a PC or laptop, a Braille display allows the user to access the computer using Braille controls and written documents are translated into Braille form. There is a special attachable machine that contains a section of small refreshable 6-dot Braille cells with movable pins in each cell (Figure 4-10). As words are printed on the screen, they are continuously transposed to Braille and the appropriate pins stick up on the pad so the user can feel the Braille symbols. There are also special printers that emboss Braille cells on heavier bond paper instead of printing typical characters with ink.

The Hal Screen Reader™ by Dolphin (Worcester, UK) is an OCR system and speech synthesizer for use with Windows operating systems. It automatically reads aloud all information on the computer screen, including its own set up and installation, with no mouse required. The FreedomBox™ software by Serotek (Minneapolis, MN) allows for voice-activated access to the Internet. It interfaces with a special Internet service provider called the FreedomBox Network. This provider is only available from voice-activated controls, not from a typical keyboard or mouse. The SARA™ from Freedom Scientific and the Ovation™ from Telesensory are portable individual OCR scanning units that convert written text directly to speech output with no visual display. Any document can be scanned and the machine reads it aloud. They also store scanned pages for future use.

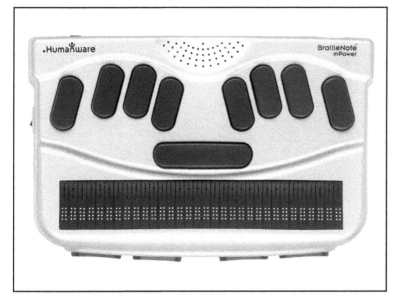

Figure 4-10. Braille-Note PK™ keyboard which allows typing in Braille format and includes a 32-cell Braille display. Documents from the computer are transposed on the refreshable Braille cells for reading by blind individuals. This model also includes a text-to-speech feature, so the Braille would mostly be used by deaf-blind individuals. (Photo courtesy of Human-Ware, Concord, CA.)

Speech Compression and Daisy Technology

Speech compression is an electronic innovation for use by low vision and blind people that allows the user to control playback speed of recorded information. The speed of the delivery of lectures or talking books can be increased without changing the auditory frequency. (In other words, one can listen at higher than normal speed and maintain the normal sound of the voice rather than listening to a high-pitched sound like the "Chipmunks.") Speech compression machines are useful for students and office workers who must process a great deal of printed and spoken material.

Between 1994 and 2000, playback technology was dramatically improved. Talking books were originally records that were played at very slow speeds of 8 or 16 rpm. Then as technology changed, they became available on audiotape as well. Now, with the introduction of digital recording, the quality and versatility of playback options has been significantly improved. A system known as DAISY (Digital Accessible Information SYstem) for the visually impaired allows listeners of digital talking books (DTBs) to do more than just alter the speed of recordings. Daisy technology allows DTBs to be produced in audio and text formats simultaneously. The text can be manipulated so the print is enlarged on a computer screen and highlighted as the audio version is played. The listener is able to start, stop, pause, navigate within passages, and skip to desired locations in the text. Some of the recordings allow the user to access a dictionary within the program to determine the meaning and pronunciation of words as well. Users can also copy materials to a clipboard for use in other formats or transfer to other computer files.

Many companies offer various types of player/recorder combinations that are compatible with Daisy technology. BookCourier™ by Springer Design (San Ramon, CA) is a small handheld MP3 player with voice recorder that allows one to download books and listen to them whenever desired. The PLEXTALK™ from Shinano Kenshi (Los Angeles, CA) is a portable version that can be attached by a USB port to a PC. When combined with the appropriate recording software, it plays in Daisy format and is compatible with MP3 audio and standard CDs as well. It can be

Figure 4-11. Victor Reader Vibe™ reads digital audio books in three versions: Daisy technology, MP3, and CD format. (Photo courtesy of HumanWare, Concord, CA.)

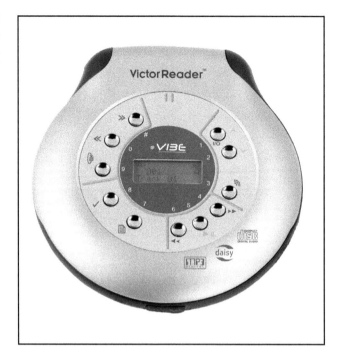

used as a CD-RW attachment to the computer as well as a playback device. Two similar handheld devices are the Telex Scholar™ and HumanWare's Victor Reader Vibe™ (Figure 4-11).

Software programs for PC such as gh PLAYER™ by gh LLC and FSReader™ by Freedom Scientific are also compatible with Daisy recordings and allow the listener to follow along with either Braille or text while controlling speed and volume.

Sometimes textbooks or other materials are unavailable in large print or recorded form. Blind or partially sighted students hire professionals or volunteers to read and record the material for them. This recording can now be done in Daisy format and replayed with a compatible playback machine. By 2008 the National Library Service for the Blind and Physically Handicapped plans to provide 20,000 titles of talking books in DTB format that can be downloaded by the user directly from a web site or through the lending library. Many thousands of books and periodicals are already available for download by those with documented visual and learning disabilities from a non-profit Internet organization called Bookshare.org. Although the organization is not for profit, there is an annual membership fee for users. (For information, contact them at www. bookshare.org.)

Since low vision electronic adaptive technology changes as quickly as any other technology, it is very important for patients to receive some guidance when purchasing a program or device. Ideally, each patient should undergo an "assistive technology assessment" by an experienced instructor before attempting to purchase a computer program for home or work use. These assessments can be scheduled through the state's agency for the blind. If there are no services available locally, the AFB has a technology center that provides reviews of the latest products and help in deciding which electronic aid may be appropriate for particular tasks. The AFB can also refer a patient to an agency in his or her local area to receive some individualized counseling. Training will improve the user's efficiency with each machine or program. The companies that market the devices often do not offer this type of training and follow-up.

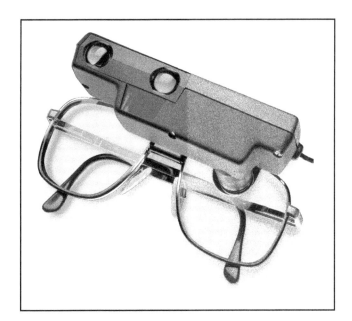

Figure 4-12. VES-AutoFocus™ telescope features bioptic telescopic lenses with an autofocus feature. (Photo courtesy of Ocutech, Chapel Hill, NC.)

Miscellaneous Electronic Devices

Electronic Telescopes

The VisAble Video Telescope™ from Betacom (Mississauga, ON, Canada) is a handheld electronic telescope that looks like a small digital camcorder. It enlarges images which the user can view through the eyepiece like a standard monocular telescope. The advantage of an electronic telescope is that it is adjustable for lower illumination settings. This eliminates one of the major problems of using a monocular telescope, which is the poor image clarity in low light conditions. The video telescope can be attached to a computer monitor and also comes with a small holder or "pod" to which it can be attached and used as a modified CCTV.

The VES-AutoFocus™ telescope system from Ocutech (Chapel Hill, NC) is a modification of conventional bioptic telescopes used for distance viewing (Figure 4-12). It has an electronic autofocus component that allows the user to change viewing distances without manually refocusing or applying a lens cap to the telescope.

Adaptive Cell Phone Programs

Programs such as ZOOMS™ and SpeechPAK TALKS™ from Nuance (Burlington, MA) and Mobile Speak™ from Optelec can be installed directly on compatible cell phones. These programs translate all text on the phone into speech so the phone can be easily used by those who cannot see the text on the phone screen. When installed, the phone verbalizes phone numbers, user menus, and calendars as well as text messages. Settings on the cell phone can be adjusted, such as the speed and pitch of the text-to-speech feature or to turn text-to-speech off for items such as key input. This type of program also allows the cell phone to be interfaced with a computer for exchange of information, like phone books, call logs, and calendar entries.

Figure 4-13. The Maestro™ from Human-Ware. A handheld computer, organizer, and email manager with Wi-Fi capabilities. (Photo courtesy of HumanWare, Concord, CA.)

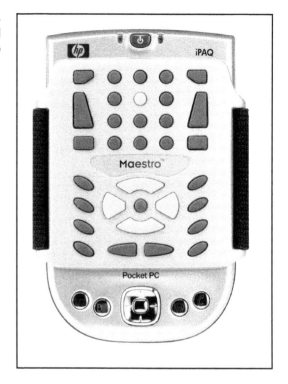

Personal Digital Assistants and Talking Organizers

The Maestro™ from HumanWare is a palm-sized computer with text-to-speech capabilities (Figure 4-13). Its features include an address book, appointment manager, calculator, MP3 player, Wi-Fi capability, and email management. It also has a choice of either a tactile QWERTY or Braille keyboard and a choice of two languages.

Parrot Voice Mate™ and VoiceNote™ by HumanWare are audio electronic organizers. These allow the user to speak directly into the machine to record addresses, phone numbers, and appointments. Numbers and information can then be retrieved with voice commands. Phone numbers can be transmitted as touch-tone signals so the numbers can be automatically dialed from a phone receiver. All information can be downloaded to a PC for other uses. BrailleNote™ is an organizer that transmits information to a refreshable Braille display rather than into synthesized speech.

Global Positioning Systems

Global positioning systems (GPS) for use by the visually impaired can be interfaced with electronic organizers. Two such systems are the Trekker™ and the BrailleNote™ GPS (both by HumanWare) (Figure 4-14). With talking menus and talking digital maps, they can be used as personal navigation systems when traveling or just when walking around unknown parts of the city. Routes can be planned and speech or Braille outputs let the user know exactly where he or she is located, including the names of buildings and cross streets. Since GPS must make contact with satellites, they do have limitations indoors and among tall buildings. Otherwise, they can be used as excellent orientation and mobility devices.

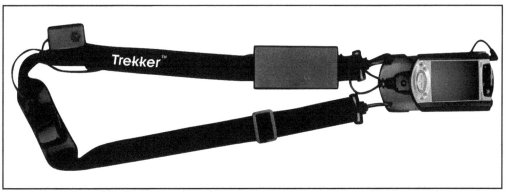

Figure 4-14. The Trekker™ GPS (with neck strap) for assistance in personal mobility. (Photo courtesy of HumanWare, Concord, CA.)

Identifiers

The Color Teller™ from Brytech (Ottawa, ON, Canada) is a portable machine that can scan clothes, pictures, and other items to determine color and tint. It can be used to match clothing or to color-code items for organization. The ColorTest Memo™ from CareTec (Vienna, Austria) is a similar device which can also be used as a stopwatch and personal calendar and to record personal memos.

The Note Teller™ from Brytech is a wallet-sized machine that scans currency to determine the denomination. It allows blind people to shop with cash, confident that they are using the correct bill to make a purchase.

Talking Calculators

Sci-Plus 300™ by HumanWare is a talking scientific calculator that includes large-print keys and a large-print screen display. It is complete with trigonometric and scientific functions for use by students and others with a need for these abilities. Also, Orbit Research (Wilmington, DE) manufactures a specially modified version of the Texas Instruments TI-34™ scientific calculator called the Orion TI-34™. Although the keys are small, each key speaks when pressed, and calculations are provided with 12-digit accuracy through the talking function, which includes a repeat option.

There are other programs for math accessibility. A good review of these can be found on the Texas School for the Blind and Visually Impaired web site (www.tsbvi.edu), which is also a good resource for many other adaptive educational materials.

Computer Attachments and Games

Key to Access™ from Premier Assistive Technology (DeWitt, MI) is a small portable flash-drive unit that can be connected to any computer with a USB port. It comes preloaded with most accessibility software and a computer user can download personal settings into it as well. Once the user's own settings are installed, when the key is attached to any computer it automatically provides access to files and settings through a floating toolbar that automatically pops up. It allows a visually impaired user to access special programs such as large print, text-to-speech word processing features, and a talking calculator without installing any additional programs to the computer's hard drive. Students or business people who use the Key are able to open their stored files at any time and place, using any compatible computer. It also provides for instant live updates of its own software technology via connecting to the Internet. Serotek has a similar item, the Key to Freedom™, and also one called PassKey™ which installs in the CD Rom drive of any computer. These two items also work with the FreedomBox Software programs for voice-activated access to computer programs and the Internet.

Standard computer games installed on Windows operating systems are not accessible for the visually impaired user, but there are other ways to log on to entertaining games. All inPlay™ is a web-based game center that offers Crazy Eights and Poker in accessible versions. BSC Games™ is another web site that offers games such as Sonic Match and Crazy Darts, which do not require vision at all. Other computer games can be purchased and installed. Chillingham™ is a whodunit adventure mystery game that does not require any vision to play. Grizzly Gulch Western Extravaganza™ is a similar interactive game that takes the player into the world of the Old West. A wide selection of accessible computer games is available through catalogue distributors of non-optical devices. See the end of Chapter 3 for addresses.

Note: The inclusion of vendors' addresses and web sites for the aids and services listed in this chapter does not imply an endorsement by the author, editors, or publisher, but is intended for informational purposes.

Web Sites and Contact Information

Ai Squared (ZoomText 9.0)
PO Box 669
Manchester Center, VT 05255
800-859-0270
www.aisquared.com

Apple (Mac OS X)
800-MY-APPLE
www.apple.com/store

Clarity (electronic magnifiers and CCTVs)
2222 Park Place, Suite 1C
Minden, NV 89423
800-575-1456
www.clarityusa.com

Freedom Scientific (OpenBook, JAWS for Windows, MAGic 9.5, SARA)
11800 31st Court N
St Petersburg, FL 33716
800-444-4443 or 727-803-8000
www.freedomscientific.com

HumanWare (PocketViewer, BrailleNote, Trekker)
175 Mason Circle
Concord, CA 94520
800-722-3393
www.humanware.com

Kurzweil Educational Systems (Kurzweil 1000, Kurzweil 3000)
100 Crosby Dr
Bedford, MA 01730
800-894-5374
www.kurzweiledu.com

NaturalSoft Ltd (NaturalReader)
#9--8680 Montcalm St
Vancouver, BC, Canada V6P 4P8
www.naturalreaders.com

Ocutech (VES-AutoFocus telescope)
109 Conner Dr, Suite 2105
Chapel Hill, NC 27514
800-326-6460
www.ocutech.com

Optelec (Supernova, Lunar, and Lunar Plus screen magnifiers)
3030 Enterprise Ct, Suite C
Vista, CA 92081
800-826-4200
www.optelec.com

Telesensory (traditional CCTVs)
www.telesensory.com *or* www.insiphil.com

Many of the devices described in this chapter are available through general distributors rather than directly from the company. If company contact information is not listed above, the device can be located through the following vendors and online stores:

- Abledata is a web site affiliated with the National Institute on Disability and Rehabilitation Research that provides information on how to contact manufacturers and distributors of all accessibility products
  www.abledata.com
- Access Ingenuity
  www.accessingenuity.com

- The American Foundation for the Blind (the **technology center** provides reviews of the latest products and help in deciding which electronic aid may be appropriate for particular tasks)
  11 Penn Plaza, Suite 300
  New York, NY 10001
  800-232-5463
  www.afb.org
- EnableMart carries items from 87 manufacturers
  www.enablemart.com
- National Association for Visually Handicapped
  www.navh.org (click on **vision aids**)
- RehabTool is a web site that will (for a fee) personally locate an item in a store near you and compare its use with other similar devices and its price among various vendors
  www.rehabtool.com
- Woodlake Technologies
  650 W Lake St, Suite 320
  Chicago, IL 60661
  800-253-4391
  www.woodlaketechnologies.com

Other Helpful Web Sites

Electronic Magnifiers and Devices

- **Clarity** (CCTVs: portable and desktop)
  www.clarityusa.com
- **Enhanced Vision** (Merlin, Max, Flipper, JORDY)
  http://enhancedvision.com
- **HumanWare** (handheld computer, Trekker, screen software, Smartview CCTVs, etc)
  www.humanware.com
- **Ocutech** (VES-AutoFocus telescopes)
  www.ocutech.com
- **Telesensory** (Pico, Olympia, Aladdin)
  www.telesensory.com

Braille and Talking Products

- **Freedom Scientific**
  www.freedomscientific.com
- **Optelec**
  www.optelec.com

Products for Computer Adaptation and Web Accessibility

- **Keyboard conversions**
  www.customkeys.com
- **Keyboards and screen magnification**
  www.sspdirect.com
- **Keyboard stickers**
  http://educationalcomputersupplies.com

Screen Magnification Software

- **Ai Squared** (ZoomText and Big Shot)
  www.aisquared.com
- **Enhanced Vision** (OpenBook and JAWS)
  www.enhancedvision.com

Text to Speech Software

- **NaturalSoft Ltd**
  www.naturalreaders.com

Clearinghouses/Miscellaneous

- **EnableMart** (vendor of electronic readers, video magnifiers, Braille adaptations)
  http://enablemart.com
- **En-Vision America** (talking prescription bottles)
  www.envisionamerica.com
- **Low Vision International** (vendor of PVO, Magnilink, ZoomText, InfoVox, Accessories)
  www.lvi.se
- **Solutions for Humans** (CCTVs, electronic magnifiers, software, screen readers, adaptive keyboards, Color Teller and Note Teller, BookCourier)
  www.sforh.com
- **Woodlake Technologies** (screen readers, note takers, Braille displays, embossers and software, speech synthesizers, screen magnifiers, more)
  www.woodlaketechnologies.com

Organizations for Accessibility Issues

- **Screen Magnifiers Homepage** (newsgroup on low vision topics and chat room for low vision patients who use screen magnification; hear from real-life users on the pros and cons of various systems)
  www.magnifiers.org
- **Web Accessibility** (Nielson Norman Group report on Web for users with disabilities)
  www.nngroup.com
- **WebAim** (simulations of what low vision patients with various diagnoses see when they are attempting to use the computer)
  www.webaim.org/simulations/lowvision

References

1. Goodrich G, Kirby J. A Comparison of patient reading performance and preference: optical devices, hand held CCTV (Innoventions Magni-Cam), or stand-mounted CCTV (Optelec Clearview or TSI Genie). *Optometry.* 2001;72:519-527.

Bibliography

Ortiz A, Chung STL, Legge GE, Jobling JT. Reading with a head-mounted video magnifier. *Optometry and Vision Science.* 1999;76:755-762.

Peterson RC, Wolffsohn JS, Rubinstein M, Lowe J. Benefits of electronic vision enhancement systems (EVES) for the visually impaired. *Am J Ophthalmol.* 2003;136:1129-1135.

Chapter 5

History Taking

KEY POINTS

- A low vision history should address rehabilitation as well as optical concerns.

- A low vision exam and history should not be attempted until the patient has reached a level of acceptance of his or her visual loss.

- A well-informed patient experiences more success with low vision aids.

- Teacher input should be solicited to determine the visual needs of school-aged patients.

Role of Patient History in Low Vision

Interpreting your patient's needs is the major challenge of low vision care and the key to future success. The only way to accurately assess the needs of individual patients is to take a thorough history. A routine history including ocular and medical conditions, family history, medications, and allergies is completed for every patient who enters an eyecare office. From this history you can ascertain many items of importance in low vision care.

The patient's ocular diagnosis provides immediate insight into the direction you may be taking. For instance, patients with macular degeneration will have central scotomas and require magnification for reading and other near tasks. Their increased need for lighting will necessitate some counseling on proper illumination. They also have a progressive disease requiring more frequent follow-up care to assess their changing needs.

The medical history provides valuable information as well (Figure 5-1). For example, insulin-dependent diabetics experience frequent fluctuations in their acuity. Several powers of low vision aids may be necessary for these patients to use as their blood sugar levels rise and fall. If they have undergone laser surgery, diabetic retinopathy patients are light sensitive and you must address their specific lighting needs. Usually they prefer more diffuse light than other visually impaired patients and will also benefit from counseling about different sunglasses and absorptive filters.

Although this routine ocular or medical history is imperative, it is not the whole story. A history for a low vision patient is more comprehensive. The four major goals are to:
1. Ascertain the visual expectations and needs of the patient
2. Determine the patient's acceptance of the visual loss and realistic understanding of the prognosis
3. Learn what social support system is in place through family, friends, or agencies
4. Create rapport and win the patient's trust

Ascertain the Visual Expectations and Needs of the Adult Patient

The visual expectations of the patient are not always realistic. For instance, a patient with severe visual loss and narrow visual field secondary to glaucoma may want to drive. When you ask what visual tasks have been given up and which are the most important to this patient, the first response will be "I want to drive again." Older people with vision loss understandably want to drive, read, play cards, and be totally independent. Moreover, they want to achieve those goals by having their vision restored to its former level. They may enter the low vision exam with unrealistic expectations. It is the job of the history taker to narrow these expectations to an achievable level.

Goals can be narrowed without discouraging the patient. For instance, if he or she desires to drive but has an acuity or visual field that apparently prohibits driving with the use of bioptics, you can say that you understand that the lack of freedom of mobility is very difficult. Don't say that they will or will not be able to drive. When asking questions, explore some other alternative mobility methods. Ask how he or she gets around at the present time. See if your patient lives near a bus route or other public transportation and whether he or she is aware of any local transportation services for senior citizens. If the patient is unaware of any local transportation, a

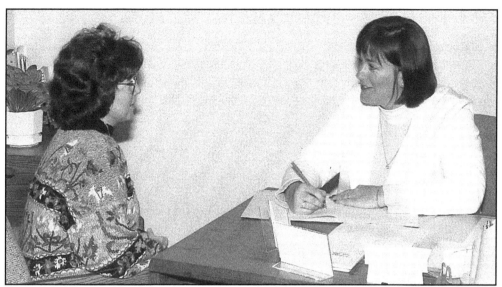

Figure 5-1. History taking helps discover the needs of the patient and also helps build a level of confidence and trust.

referral to a social agency will be in order. Sometimes patients have a fear of becoming lost if they use public transportation because they cannot see well enough to read bus schedules, maps, or the signs on bus stops. Sometimes the inability to read a watch might inhibit a person from using buses for fear of missing the scheduled pickup and becoming stranded. A handheld telescope and a mobility lesson concerning bus routes might relieve the first fear, while a talking or large-print watch would relieve the second.

Conversely, low vision patients may have their expectations set too low. They may have tried a magnifier in the past without success and feel sure that you cannot help them in any way. They are frequently unaware of services and aids that are available. It is necessary for the person taking the history to ask leading questions about specific vocational needs or hobbies. Also inquire about requirements for distance viewing other than driving and activities of daily living that have become difficult. You might question what usually is eaten for dinner, how it is cooked or prepared, what problems arise in using the stove, and how grocery shopping is done. Some patients eat cold cereal and packaged food because of an inability to see the dials on the stove or fear of starting a fire. Marking the stove dials with bump-ons (tactile dots) to locate various temperature settings can remedy this problem. Grocery shopping may be done at the local convenience store because of an inability to travel to the supermarket or to maneuver in a large store. Providing the names of grocery stores who deliver or those who have shoppers' helpers on staff may change the patient's diet and health.

Only when you have gained a thorough understanding of the patient's true needs can you be successful in improving his or her adjustment to visual loss. A good low vision clinic will address these social or rehabilitation concerns as well as optical needs. Asking appropriate questions will direct you toward success with the first aid chosen instead of trying magnifiers haphazardly. A patient who wants to see piano music will not benefit from a handheld magnifier. Both hands must be free to play the music. The same is true of those who love crossword puzzles. Hand magnifiers may be better than high power spectacles, however, for reading recipes while cooking.

Questions to Narrow a Patient's Needs

Chief Complaint
- What is the main problem you have related to your visual loss?
- What visual struggle affects you the most in your daily life?
- If we can restore one task for you with the help of aids, what do you most want it to be?

Vocational
- What is your job?
- What difficulties have you been experiencing in your work because of your eye problem?
- What size print do you most often encounter in your work?
- Do you have distance limitations such as working at a computer screen or a large drafting table? Have you measured this viewing distance?

General
- Have you used magnifiers in the past? Were they helpful? Why or why not? How do you think we could improve on them for your use?
- What kind of light do you use for reading?
- What light is best for you?
- Do you experience glare outdoors or difficulty adjusting to light changes?

Hobbies
- Have you had to give up any hobbies or sports specifically because of your visual loss?
- Does your vision prevent you from trying some sport or hobby you would like to try?

Activities of Daily Living
- Do you drive? If not, what method of transportation do you use?
- Do you have someone you can rely on to take you on important trips, like grocery shopping and doctor appointments? Do you have someone you can rely on for simple trips like visits to the library?
- Can you see the labels and price tags when you shop?
- Do you cook your own food? What is your biggest difficulty in preparing meals? Has your menu changed since your vision has become poorer?
- Do you feel you can keep your house clean and finish the laundry or are you having trouble with household chores?
- Can you read your own mail?
- Do you write your own checks and balance your checkbook easily, or do you find it difficult?

 # Determine Level of Acceptance of Visual Loss

Sometimes patients receive low vision care too soon or at the request of a family member instead of from self-motivation. People come to ophthalmology exams with high expectations of cures and fears of blindness. When presented with the news that nothing can be done medically, they may be overwhelmed with grief and dread. It will take some time for these strong reactions to evolve into a search for rehabilitation or an acceptance of the condition. The patient will forget anything you say about low vision or rehabilitation at the outset and often will reject it. The time it takes a particular patient to accept the need for help will vary depending on personality, age, and family support.

Another common misinterpretation that a patient may bring to the low vision evaluation is a misunderstanding of his or her diagnosis and prognosis. Ophthalmologists like to cure blindness and perform surgery. They are not happy when there is no cure available and sometimes unintentionally fail to discuss the subject with patients. If a patient is told to keep returning for follow-up, the impression may be that there will be some improvement or that a treatment is on the horizon. There may also be a failure to understand the diagnosis itself because of lack of explanation. (If you discover that a patient has a poor understanding of his or her diagnosis and unrealistic expectations about the prognosis, you should inform the ophthalmologist or social worker involved so they can help the patient come to terms with the situation.)

What the Patient Needs to Know

- In this office we care about you.

- The questions you are being asked are not meant to pry. We want to be aware of your difficulties so we can better serve you.

- We can show you optical devices to help with reading or distance vision. Your vision will not be as good as it used to be, but it can be better than it is at present.

- There are rehabilitation personnel readily available to help you with adjustment to both the physical and emotional difficulties of your visual loss.

During the low vision history, ask the patient (not a family member) to explain to you what is wrong with his or her eyes. Ask if the problem is expected to improve or worsen and what this means for his or her future. It is not the job of the assistant to provide the patient with the truth or discuss the prognosis, but the information will allow you to determine how much motivation the patient has to work with low vision aids (and their inherent problems). If Mr. Jones thinks laser surgery is going to cure his eyes next month, he will not spend money on computerized optical devices. He also may not devote energy to practice reading at a very close reading distance. The well-informed patient who has accepted the visual loss is the patient who will be most successful with low vision aids.

Questions to Evaluate Acceptance

- What medically is wrong with your eyes?
- Is your vision going to get better? Worse?
- Is your doctor still considering any treatments?
- Do you feel that your vision problem has been thoroughly explained to you? Do you understand it?

Determine Level of Support of Family, Friends, and Agencies

A visually impaired person is disabled. Because a low vision exam is often the stepping stone to rehabilitation, it is important to assess the type of support your patient receives at home. Elderly low vision patients may not have a spouse or other family member who can drive or offer assistance in the normal activities of daily living. These patients, and those who live alone, will require more extensive help and referrals to social service agencies. Other seniors may live in an assisted-living facility and have most of these activities taken care of by the staff of the organization. They are luckier and may do very nicely with just a magnifier and a subscription to a large-print newspaper. (Be sure to contact the social worker at the assisted-living facility to help coordinate services.)

A loss of sight robs a person of independence. Some dependencies are obvious, such as the inability to drive. There are other losses that are more subtle and personal, and can be even more devastating. As reading ability diminishes, private correspondence can no longer be private. A third person is necessary to read the mail. Personal financial records must be shared with others in order to write checks and balance accounts. This makes people feel very vulnerable. Because of these very personal needs it is vital that each low vision patient have the help of someone he or she can trust. If there is no family support or close friend, a social service agency or other professionals should become involved. A referral to a social worker is indicated.

If there is a good family network, write down the name and phone number of the relative who comes to the low vision evaluation. This person will be a good contact if any confusion arises. When training the patient in the use of low vision aids, ask one or more supportive family members to be present. Then if a problem arises at home, at least two people will be trained correctly, eliminating a need to call you for help.

Questions to Determine Support Level

- Who brought you to the exam today? Are they friends or relatives?
- Who do you call if you need help with shopping or other chores?
- Do you have people whom you can trust and rely on for personal needs such as balancing your accounts?
- Do you live with or near people who can help you on a daily basis? (Unless the patient offers the information, do not ask if he or she lives alone. Some elderly people do not like to give out this information for security reasons.)

Create Rapport and Win Trust

As you may realize by now, low vision is a very personal matter. It challenges a patient's independence and sense of dignity. There are many fears and frustrations involved. During past medical exams, however, doctors may have been business-like, addressing only medical concerns. Patients learn to keep private matters to themselves. Although you seem interested, most patients will not divulge their personal fears or desires suddenly. They will explain gladly what they want to read, because they have been doing that since presbyopia affected them. It is socially acceptable to have difficulties reading the newspaper. The deeper concerns of patients may take a few visits to emerge, as you win their trust. By asking questions during the history, a dialogue occurs that will hopefully help the patient feel at ease and realize that personal issues are going to be addressed.

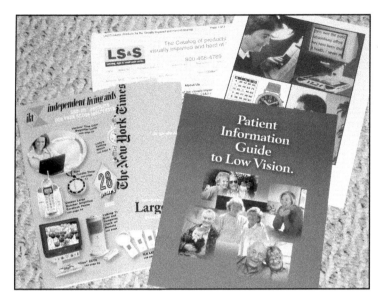

Figure 5-2. A sample of patient education materials to provide at the first visit.

To help create this rapport as quickly as possible, educate your patients. Give a non-optical aids catalogue to every low vision patient on the first visit. Talk about other people who have been helped in hobbies or vocations. Use anecdotes to explain what types of aids and agencies are available. A patient who does not know what is available will not understand how to seek help.

This may not sound like history taking, but is necessary for a successful low vision exam. Only after the patient is educated will he or she be able to give proper responses to questions regarding low vision history. On the other hand, it is important not to overeducate on the first visit. Patients who are nervous about visual loss are not going to retain very much information. For that reason, the history may evolve over the course of the exam or after several follow-up visits. Do not blindly stick to goals set at the outset, because the patient's needs and expectations may change as he or she realizes possibilities or experiences frustration.

To educate your patients, create a packet of information to present to everyone during the initial visit (Figure 5-2). This will ensure that even if Mrs. Smith does not return for follow-up, information is in her possession to allow her to seek care on her own time. Collect pertinent materials in advance in large quantities. Then place these materials in large envelopes or files to present to your patients. Such a packet might include:

- A list of local and national social service agencies offering help to visually impaired people. This may include optical help, social groups, support or advocacy organizations, banks that offer large-print checks to customers, and grocery stores that deliver or offer shopping assistance to disabled customers.
- A non-optical aids catalogue such as that from Independent Living Aids or Maxi-Aids.
- A brochure from the American Academy of Ophthalmology or American Optometric Association about low vision care.
- A handout listing other publications that may be helpful to the patient such as information and an application form from the National Library Service for the Blind and Physically Handicapped and information from the National Association for Visually Handicapped.
- A large-print calling card listing the name of your clinic, the hours of operation, the person to contact with concerns or questions, and the phone number.

The contact information for each of these agencies and groups can be found in Chapters 2, 3, and 9.

Figure 5-3. Children prefer to read at very close distances rather than use magnifiers.

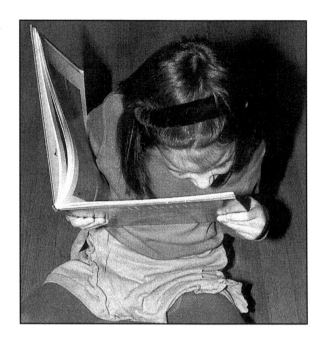

History Taking for the Pediatric Low Vision Patient

The low vision needs of children are different from those of adults. Many topics already discussed pertain to children, such as ocular and medical history, social support, and lack of independence. Family history of progressive diseases is very important also. That information will help determine the type of follow-up and social service intervention that may be necessary. The real difference in the history of a child, however, is in assessing the optical needs.

The major visual task of children is to see in school. Because of this, the teacher should be as involved in the low vision history as the parents. Teachers usually are willing to attend a low vision evaluation or at least to discuss the visual demands of their classroom over the phone. Teacher input is very important in deciding which aid to prescribe for a child. The parents alone usually are unaware of all the child's specific visual needs. A phone call to the school is done easily when scheduling a low vision appointment and has great potential benefit.

Children have large reserves of accommodative ability and can see print at near in spite of visual loss. They simply hold the material close and their accommodation acts as a built-in low vision aid (Figure 5-3). Although this eliminates the need for constant use of a magnifier for near, it should not preclude the prescription of one. Constant use of the full power of accommodation can fatigue the eyes, causing a lack of desire to read. A supplementary magnifier can help make reading more satisfying and comfortable. Electronic reading machines and software programs that enlarge print are very important for school-aged children. While taking the history, ask about computer use. Is the child already using a computer? Is he or she able to use most standard programs and games? If the child has not been successful in the use of computers, an assistive technology assessment is indicated and will usually be provided by the state agency for the blind or by the school system.

Telescopes for distance viewing are good even for young children. They can be used in the classroom for board work, in the stands of a ball field to view sports, in auditoriums and movies to enjoy theater events, and to read signs and bus route numbers to facilitate independent mobility.

It is possible to prescribe telescopes at an early age, including preschool and kindergarten. This gives the child an awareness of distance, and the telescope becomes a regular part of the viewing habits while there is no stigma involved. If presented with a telescope in the later grades, social pressure usually makes it difficult to use them regularly and confidently.

Because children play hard it is imperative that they wear safety glasses. No matter what type of glasses are prescribed, the lenses should be polycarbonate and the frames should be sturdy enough to withstand strong forces. For sports with potential eye contact by a ball or racquet, frames should pass the American National Standards Institute Z87.1 safety standards updated in 2003. For low vision children this cannot be emphasized enough. Children are more prone to accidents as a result of their visual disability and have more to lose if they sustain further damage to their eyes.

As with all learning disabilities, the parents of the child must advocate for services for their child. As one of the primary contacts with the vision system, it is important for the ophthalmology office to mention this to parents. Many of them assume incorrectly that just because their child has a disability that they will automatically receive services. The parents should be encouraged to ask for low vision aids, a technology assessment, and help from a special educator specifically trained in the needs of children with visual disabilities. The parent should contact the school department as well as the state agency for the blind if he or she has not already done so.

Questions for the Pediatric Low Vision History

(Ask these questions of the child, the parent[s], and the teacher.)

- What activities is the child involved in that are limited by vision? Does he or she play a musical instrument? Is the child able to play games with siblings or friends? Can the TV be seen successfully?
- How far does the child sit from the board or other distant objects in the classroom (such as the clock)?
- Is he or she able to read the appropriate size of printed material without much difficulty? What print size generally is used in the classroom?
- Is there a vision resource room or itinerant vision teacher available at the school?
- Does he or she engage in any sports or extracurricular activities that require better vision?
- Has there been a desire to participate in any activities that were not tried because of the visual limitations?
- How does he or she get to and from school? Can the child move freely about the school without assistance?
- How close are books held to the eyes when reading? Does the child complain of headaches after long-term near work?
- What type of lighting is used for reading?
- Are current glasses made with polycarbonate lenses? Even if there is no distance refractive error, are safety glasses worn?
- Has a telescope or other magnifier ever been tried?

Low vision history taking may sound involved, but it need not be tedious in actual practice. This thorough discussion is to help you understand why you are taking a history and some issues to consider. The actual questioning should only take several minutes. With practice you will become quite proficient at recognizing which questions to ask for a given situation. The following is a suggested form for taking a low vision history, to guide you in your investigation of each patient's needs.

Low Vision History

Date of visit:
Patient name:
Phone number:
Age of patient:
Name and phone of support person (and teacher if applicable):

Ocular diagnosis:
Prognosis for vision:
Visual field loss:
Ocular history:
Medical history:
Current medications:
Allergies:
Patient's primary goal(s):
Distance needs:

Near needs:

Preferred lighting:

Magnifiers previously used and problems encountered:

Vocation:

Grade in school, name of school, name of teacher:

Hobbies:

Limited activities of daily living:
     Shopping/cooking:
     Grooming:
     Housekeeping:
     Correspondence/money management:

Method of travel/mobility:

Level of understanding diagnosis/prognosis:

Living arrangements:

Wearing polycarbonate safety lenses?

Chapter 6

Assessment of Visual Function

KEY POINTS

- Move the test chart closer to allow the patient to experience success in reading more letters and for a more precise evaluation of distance acuity. Record the actual testing distance.

- Always verify the refractometric measurement before beginning low vision testing. Optimal refractive correction is imperative.

- Near vision should be tested using continuous text cards and selecting the smallest size of print that can be read fluently.

Distance Acuity Testing

Traditional methods of testing acuity are not practical for low vision patients. Once acuity has dropped below 20/80 there are only a few optotypes (letters, numbers, or other symbols) per line on the most commonly used distance test charts. These optotypes are usually variations of E, with one or two others that can be easily memorized. This lack of choice causes inaccurate testing; recorded acuity reflects patient memory more than functional visual ability. Projected charts have the added problem of glare and can only be used in dim light. Coupled with variability in bulb strength and the condition and color of the projection screen, this can seriously affect the contrast of the letters against the background, therefore artificially creating a false test of contrast sensitivity as well as acuity. Psychologically, if someone can only see the largest letters on a chart there may be a feeling of hopelessness and fear. Practically, if the patient only reads the 20/400 E, it does not allow the examiner to gain an accurate understanding of visual limitations and abilities.

There are other problems in assessing acuity using traditional Snellen projector charts. Each line includes a varying *number* of optotypes, thereby changing the validity of test results using different sizes. If one line contains only one letter and it is seen correctly, but the following line has four letters where only one is seen correctly, it does not really determine which of the lines represents the true acuity level. Also, there is not a uniform difference in size between the various lines. The increase in size of optotypes from one line to another is only about 25% in the lower lines, while the larger letters increase in size by as much as 100% between lines. Another lack of uniformity is the distance between letters per line. Smaller letters are affected by crowding, while the larger letters are not because there is more space between each figure.

Distance test charts specifically designed for low vision testing alleviate these problems. Most of these charts are handheld rather than projected. They can be used in any lighting condition to better duplicate the normal situation of each patient. Most of the charts have optotypes that correspond to finer gradations of acuity between 20/80 and 20/800. For instance, there are letters that correlate to 20/120, 20/140, 20/160, and 20/180. Each line contains several characters so memorization is less likely.

Low vision test charts come in many varieties. The preferred charts are those that eliminate all of the problems associated with projected Snellen charts. The most commonly used are those based on the Ferris-Bailey chart that was used in the Early Treatment Diabetic Retinopathy Study (ETDRS). These charts have an equal number of letters per line with equal spacing between the letters so that each line represents a testing situation equivalent to all other lines. The increase of type size is also uniform and based on a logarithmic progression where letters double in size every three rows. To record the visual resolution of letters on a particular line a different notation is used. This notation is referred to as logMAR (logarithm of the Minimum Angle of Resolution). The test is designed to be used at a distance of 4 meters and the letters are calibrated appropriately for resolution at that distance. The largest letters give a score of 1.0 (which corresponds to 20/200 Snellen equivalent if testing at 4 meters) and each line below that gives a score of 0.1 less. Most charts used in low vision are calibrated with both logMAR notation and Snellen equivalents for easy conversion. (See Table 6-1 for a comparison chart.) If the chart is moved closer to the patient, relative distance magnification results and accurate testing of very low acuity is possible.

LogMAR charts are preferred in most low vision testing situations because of the inherent accuracy and reproducibility. Other charts have Sloan letters or the letters H,O,T,V. (Sloan

Table 6-1
Log and Snellen Acuity Comparisons

logMAR Acuity	Snellen Equivalent (when tested at 4M)
-0.3	20/10
-0.2	20/12.5
-0.1	20/16
0.0	20/20
0.1	20/25
0.2	20/32
0.3	20/40
0.4	20/50
0.5	20/70
0.6	20/80
0.7	20/100
0.8	20/125
0.9	20/160
1.0	20/200

letters are similar to Snellen letters but are calibrated in meter equivalents called M units. For further discussion on M units see the section on near vision testing.)

Still other distance vision tests have optotypes designed for pediatric and illiterate use. The most common of these is the Lea symbols chart (Figure 6-1) which has representations of a house, an apple, a square, and a circle. Other illiterate test charts use numbers or Landolt Cs, which are rings with a small break in the circumference. The patient is directed to say whether the break is on the left, right, top, or bottom. Some of these charts are handheld and others are designed to fit into an illuminated stand on a rolling base for ease in changing testing distances (Figure 6-2). When brought closer, the size of the print enlarges in a reciprocal relationship. If you bring the chart forward to one quarter the distance (eg, 5 feet instead of 20 feet), the print is magnified four times. In this way, it is possible to measure acuity accurately when it is as low as 20/800 because a "200" size letter becomes an "800" size. In log notation, each time you halve the reading distance a doubling of size occurs, allowing acuity testing with optotypes three lines lower on the chart. This eliminates the need to record acuity as simply "hand motions" or "counts fingers" when the vision is severely limited.

Another popular test chart for low vision is Feinbloom Distance Test Chart for the Partially Sighted (Figure 6-3). This is a handheld flip chart that has much larger letters and can be used to assess vision as low as 20/2800 when held at a distance of 5 feet. The problem with this chart is that it still contains some of the difficulties of the old testing methods such as few letters per line and no variability in the letters presented at various sizes. The Colenbrander Low Vision Chart (Figure 6-4) is designed for severely impaired patients and is to be used at a distance of 1 meter. It uses numbers instead of letters, so it can be used with children or adults who do not read English characters. It tests vision as low as 20/1000. There are other types of handheld charts available for low vision use, but many of them are becoming obsolete with the advent of logMAR testing.

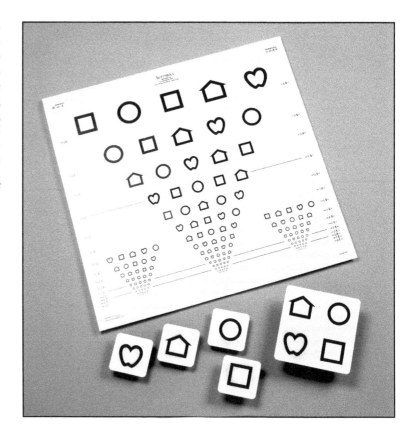

Accurate acuity testing gives us the ability to assess magnification needs more clearly. For instance, a patient with 20/200 acuity needs 10 D of magnification to read small print. Only 6 D are needed by the patient with 20/120 acuity. Using a traditional Snellen chart, since the patient would not be able to read any letters on the 20/100 line, the acuity would be recorded as 20/200 and the magnification would be overprescribed, actually reducing the usable field of view. Patients also gain confidence when they can see many letters. Some patients often remark that this is the first time in a long while that they can read the chart. This starts the low vision exam on a positive note and encourages further success.

Changing testing distances requires recalculation of acuity. On a chart designed for 20-foot testing distances, the optotype that corresponds to 20/200 acuity is 87 mm tall and subtends an angle of 50 minutes of arc on the retina. When testing the visual acuity of low vision patients, if the chart is moved forward, the testing distance and retinal image size have a reciprocal relationship. For instance, if you test the vision at 10 feet, which is 1/2 the usual testing distance, the retinal image size is doubled (2/1). If the testing distance is moved even closer, to 5 feet, the retinal image size is quadrupled (4/1) since this testing distance is one fourth (1/4) of the standard 20 feet.

Although the testing distance may be changed, the optotype obviously remains the same size. In the example above, if testing at a distance of 10 feet with an optotype that is still a 200-foot number (87 mm high), the acuity is recorded as 10/200 which is proportional and equivalent to an acuity of 20/400 (10/200 x 2/2 = 20/400). If vision is tested at 5 feet, the acuity should be recorded as 5/200, which is equivalent to 20/800 (5/200 x 4/4 = 20/800). Even when we test acuity using log charts, it is still customary to record the acuity in Snellen equivalents

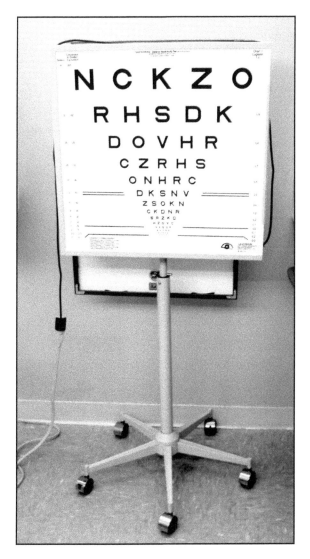

Figure 6-2. The Lighthouse Distance Visual Acuity Test designed for a 4-meter testing distance. Lines are recorded in Snellen, logMAR, and metric notations to help simplify conversions. The rolling stand makes it easy to vary testing distances.

as well. Record acuity with the actual testing distance in the numerator and the optotype size in the denominator. Do not convert to "20" equivalents before recording. For example, if vision is tested at 5 feet and the 100-size letters are read clearly, vision is recorded as 5/100, not as 20/400. This allows future examiners to duplicate the same testing standards.

Since most log charts are designed to be used at a distance of 4 meters, be sure to record if the acuity was tested at a closer range. Record the testing distance after the log units. For example, under normal conditions 0.9 log correlates to 20/160 Snellen acuity. If the chart is moved forward to 2 meters and the patient's BCVA is 0.9 log it represents 20/320 Snellen acuity. This could be recorded as 0.9 log @ 2 meters.

However, logMAR acuity notation does not share a reciprocal relationship with distance like Snellen notation. For example, if you move a Snellen chart to half the distance, you would double the Snellen acuity (20/160 at 10 feet would become 10/160 which is the equivalent of 20/320). If you mistakenly doubled the *log acuity* to 1.8 instead of 0.9, you would be misrepresenting the acuity as approximately 20/1200. This is because a change of only 0.3 logMAR

Figure 6-3. The Fein-bloom Distance Test Chart for the Partially Sighted™ is a handheld distance acuity test. Visual acuity as low as 20/2800 can be recorded when used at a distance of 5 feet. (Photo courtesy of Eschenbach Optik of America, Ridgefield, CT.)

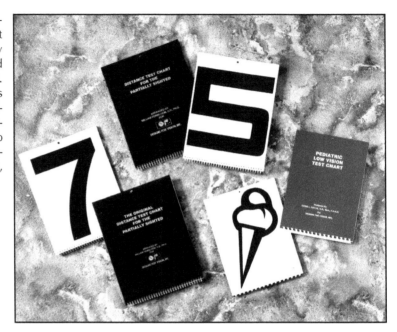

Figure 6-4. Lea numbers can also be used for those who cannot read English characters. This Colenbrander test chart is designed for a testing distance of 1 meter, which can be kept constant using the attached cord. This chart measures visual acuity as low as 20/1000. (Photo courtesy of Good-Lite, Elgin, IL.)

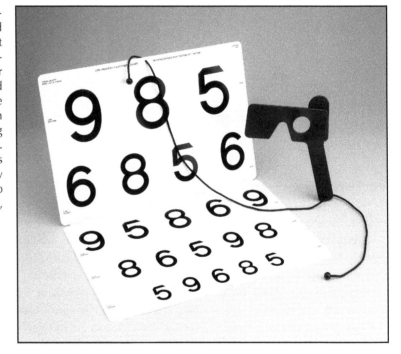

already represents a doubling of acuity. So when the chart is moved to a 2-meter testing distance, instead of doubling the log acuity measure, just add 0.3. If the chart is moved to a 1-meter testing distance, add 0.6. For example, 0.7 log acuity when measured at 4 meters is equivalent to 20/100 Snellen. If 0.7 log is measured at 2 meters, convert for the distance by adding 0.3, so the measured acuity is 1.0 log (0.7 + 0.3) or 20/200. If 0.7 log acuity is measured

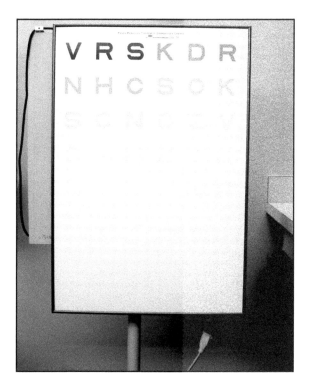

Figure 6-5. The Pelli-Robson Contrast Sensitivity Chart helps with the accurate assessment of contrast resolution and can help with the determination of lens power and illumination levels.

at 1 meter, convert by adding 0.6, so the actual measured acuity is 1.3 log (0.7 + 0.6) which represents a 20/400 Snellen equivalent. In summary, when recording vision with log charts, do not try to create equivalencies by multiplication. Because of this discrepancy, it is always a good idea to record acuity in Snellen equivalents after recording the log acuity in order to avoid mistakes.

All patients should be examined first in daylight conditions. Ideally, also test office and retail workers under fluorescent lights. Specific lighting for other professions or avocations should be duplicated when possible to determine the patient's functional ability in his or her normal environment.

In addition to standard distance acuity, it is important to test the contrast sensitivity of patients. When patients have decreased vision, they are very sensitive to changes in the contrast of objects they are viewing. It is much easier to see the black letters of a test chart against a stark white background than it is to see the contours of a face or dark items in shadow. Since most of real life takes place in a lower contrast world, contrast sensitivity should be tested as well as acuity as a routine part of a low vision exam.

The Pelli-Robson chart (Figure 6-5) is an easy way to test contrast sensitivity since it looks similar to a distance acuity chart. It is also arranged in logarithmic progression like the logMAR acuity charts, but here the log units of change refer to the level of contrast between lines, not the size of the type. In fact, all optotypes are the same size and spacing, so the only change from line to line is the contrast. The test is performed at 1 meter and the sensitivity is recorded in log units. A higher score indicates better contrast acuity. A poor performance on this test will indicate a need for higher levels of magnification or for stronger lighting for most tasks.

Contrast acuity is affected by dim illumination, but also by excessive glare. Because of this, glare testing is also indicated for many low vision patients. Those with ocular albinism or diabetic

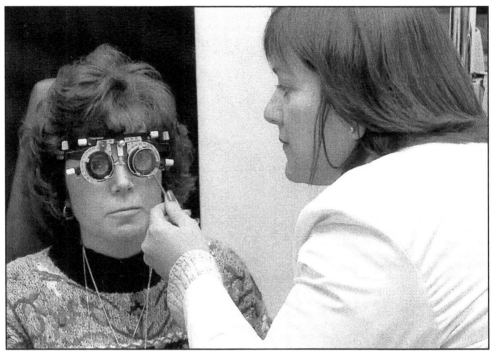

Figure 6-6. Refractometry using a trial frame and loose lenses. The handheld cross cylinder power is chosen using the patient's just noticeable difference.

retinopathy are sensitive to bright light, while those with retinitis pigmentosa cannot function well in low light and experience delays in their ability to adapt from a lighted area to one of darkness. Patients may also have cataracts that have not been removed because of a poor visual prognosis. The glare associated with cataracts may exacerbate the vision loss from the patient's primary pathology. For example, if a patient with macular degeneration has a visual acuity of 20/80 and a cataract develops, the vision may deteriorate to a level of 20/120 or worse and become even more limited than this due to glare. Contrast sensitivity and glare testing will not diagnose these conditions, but can provide clues to functional problems. Counseling about lighting and absorptive filters can then be customized for patients' individual needs.

Verifying Refractive Error

Never assume that a patient is wearing his or her best refractive correction. Frequently retinal surgeons have followed these patients for laser or other surgical treatments, and the health of the retina has been their priority. It may have been several years since the glasses were updated. In other cases, functional low vision problems may simply be overlooked refraction problems such as uncorrected high astigmatism. Each patient deserves thorough and accurate refractometry before low vision testing. This should be performed by the refractive expert in your office.

Low vision refractometric measurements are best performed "the old-fashioned way," using a trial frame and loose lenses (Figure 6-6). A phoropter may be helpful during initial retinoscopy for convenience of the examiner, but the small visual apertures of the refractor limit the field of view. Patients with central scotomas have better acuity from a retinal point that is peripheral to the macula. The *eccentric view* and head position necessary to use this peripheral point will be impossible to achieve while using a refractor. Use a trial frame for refinement and vision evaluation. The best trial lenses to use for low vision are the full aperture lenses with a thin metal carrier. The lenses with wide red or black edges provide very small visual apertures, especially in the higher powers, and are no improvement over the refractor. The acuity chart should be located at a distance of 10 feet or even 5 feet, as in the initial acuity testing. Cylindrical correction should be determined with the use of a handheld Jackson cross cylinder as well, since they are available in powers of ±0.25, ±0.50, and ±1.00.

Before refining cylinder or sphere it is necessary to detect the weakest lens that causes a noticeable difference in vision by the patient. Try ±0.50 and ±1.00 D lenses, increasing to ±2.00 D or higher as necessary until the patient is aware of a subjective decrease in visual resolution when the lens is applied. This "just noticeable difference" (JND) will determine the power of lens that will be used during subjective refinement during refractometry. For example, if a patient has a JND of 1.00 D and retinoscopy reveals a refractive error of +3.00, instead of flipping ±0.25 D lenses in the phoropter during refractometry, increments of +1.00 should be introduced as the choices when asking a patient if the vision is better through "lens one or lens two." Similarly, a cross cylinder of ±1.00 D should be used for refining cylinder. Some practitioners correlate JND with the denominator of the acuity: 20/100 has a 1.00 D JND, 20/200 has a 2.00 D JND, etc.[1] In addition, if a patient has less astigmatic error than the JND, it is not necessary to provide a cylinder correction. For instance, if a patient has a 0.50 D cylinder error, but his or her JND is 1.50 D, the correction of astigmatism is not necessary. The spherical equivalent of this lens is only 0.25 so will not be noticed if it is missing. The spherical correction can be employed and the difference will not affect the functional visual ability.

Low vision refractometry is not routine, and some special techniques may need to be attempted. A plano contact lens may be used for smoothing irregular corneal surfaces to provide the best refractive correction. The stenopaic slit and other "old-fashioned" devices may also prove helpful. Keratometry prior to refractometry may give clues about astigmatism. A refractometrist needs to be creative to find the optimum correction under less than optimum conditions.

What the Patient Needs to Know

- Please do not guess at letters on the chart. We would like to know the level of print that is comfortable for you to read.

- When we check you for a glasses prescription and "lens number one" looks the same as "lens number two," tell the examiner. You will not always notice a difference, and that is okay.

Finally, remember that the measurement is being done at a distance closer than 20 feet. The final distance prescription will be focused for 5 feet or 10 feet (wherever the chart is being held). Remove up to 0.50 D of plus power to convert it to focus for optical infinity.

Near Vision Testing

Traditionally, ophthalmic and optometric assistants are taught to encourage patients to guess and struggle when testing acuity. Acuity is recorded as the absolute maximum number of letters that are guessed correctly. Because low vision is concerned with functional visual ability, the technique is different. If someone can identify individual letters of a given size, it does not necessarily correlate to reading ability. When determining the functional ability of a patient for low vision aids, not only acuity is considered, but also literacy, accuracy, reading rate, reading comprehension, and endurance.[2] For this reason, the size of print necessary for fluent reading is often considerably larger. In low vision, we record near acuity as the smallest size of print that can be read *fluently and easily*. When a patient begins to struggle with print, it is too small. Discontinue testing and record the previous, larger size print as the acuity level.

Perform near testing at two distances. First, allow the patient to read at his or her preferred distance. Measure and record the eye-to-print distance as well as the size of the print. This can be done with both eyes open. Allow the patient to use current reading glasses or magnifiers, remove distance correction, or use any other preferred method to see the near target. The goal here is to assess the current reading ability. Low vision aids that cannot improve on this level will not be accepted. No matter how scientific your measurements or logical your selection, an aid has to give the patient some functional advantage or it will not be used. Also, it will give you information on reading distances that feel natural or comfortable to the patient.

Second, measure the functional reading ability for each eye alone at a distance of 40 cm. This should be performed while the patient is corrected optically to emmetropia and with an additional +2.50 add in the trial frame or attached to accurate distance spectacles with Halberg clips. This combination provides optimal focus without magnification at the 40 cm distance. This test will be used to calculate the power of magnification necessary for near tasks. Because improved visual function at near is the goal of most low vision aids, accuracy in testing is very important. The 40 cm distance must be kept constant and the optical correction must be optimum.

When testing near acuity, use reading cards that are specifically designed for low vision. Since testing is performed at a 40 cm reading distance, many cards have a 40 cm long cord attached for ease in regulating the testing distance. These near tests include miniature versions of the log charts (Figure 6-7), reading cards that include individual words (like the Lighthouse "Game" card), the Fonda-Anderson Plastic Reading Card, and continuous text reading cards (Figure 6-8). A preferred low vision near test is the MN Read Test (Minnesota Low Vision Reading Test, Optelec, Vista, CA). It consists of continuous text cards that can be used to evaluate reading speed as well as near acuity. This helps to determine a "critical print size" which is the minimum size of print that still allows the maximum reading speed.

MN Read cards contain print that is measured on the log scale and are available from -0.5 to 1.3 log when tested at 40 cm. Each card contains 10 words, all of the same print size, with a total of 60 characters. Once acuity is measured as it is with any standard continuous text card, reading speed can also be timed using the preferred print size.

Other reading cards are calibrated in meter equivalents (M units) instead of log, Jaeger, or point size. M units were devised by Dr. Louise Sloan to simplify calculations of magnification.[3] Letters that subtend a 5′ angle on the retina when viewed at a distance of 1 meter are called 1M print. A 2M letter subtends the same 5′ retinal angle when viewed at a distance of 2 meters, 3M at 3 meters, etc.

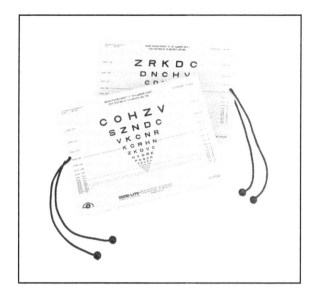

Figure 6-7. The logMAR system of acuity measurement is also used on near charts that are designed for a testing distance of 40 cm. The attached cord helps maintain an accurate reading distance. (Photo courtesy of Good-Lite, Elgin, IL.)

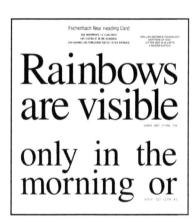

Figure 6-8. Continuous text near reading cards help determine if a patient is able to read an unbroken line of print rather than just isolated letters. (Photo courtesy of Eschenbach Optik of America, Ridgefield, CT.)

This 5′ angle is the same size as that which projects on the retina from a "20" size letter on a Snellen chart at 20 feet. In terms of visual acuity, 1M at 1 meter and 20/20 are equivalent. The difference is that M units are calibrated in meters as is dioptric power. Because a 1 D lens has a focal length of 1 meter, there is a direct correlation between M units and diopters. This makes it easy to determine powers of magnification necessary for good reading ability. The only thing to remember is that reading cards generally have very high contrast print and therefore predict a better acuity with a particular power of magnification. In reality, when reading newspapers and other low contrast texts, most people will require a higher magnification to achieve the same reading success that was achieved with a high contrast near reading card.

Record near acuity as a ratio. The reading distance in centimeters is the numerator. The print size in M units or log notation is the denominator. For example, 40/4M means the patient can read 4M print held at a distance of 40 cm. Remember to record the acuity where the reading is fluent, not where it is difficult. When measuring using a log chart, record as a ratio or just as a log acuity at 40 cm (40/0.7 log or 0.7 log @ 40 cm).

In some cases there is a discrepancy of more than two lines between the acuity of the two eyes when tested at the same distance. In this case, the better seeing eye alone can be corrected by low vision aids. The power of the aid will be selected according to the acuity of this stronger eye. In high powers of magnification, patients use only one eye at a time anyway, so monocular correction will not be debilitating. If there is some interference from the eye with poorer vision, an occluder can be worn over that eye or the final near prescription can incorporate a frosted lens on that side. For temporary occlusion, opaque press-on filters may be applied to the lens of the nonpreferred eye and removed after the near task is completed.

Visual Fields and Low Vision

Many types of visual field loss affect the functional ability of patients in different ways. Central scotomas can eliminate the ability to recognize faces, read print, or see straight ahead. To cope, the patient must use magnification and adopt an unusual head or eye position, known as eccentric viewing, which allows him or her to use an off-center yet visually healthier portion of the retina for seeing. Altitudinal defects occur with glaucoma or optic neuritis. These defects block the lower or upper portion of the visual field. When the defect is in the superior field, the patient is in danger of walking into overhangs or other objects such as tree limbs that might strike the upper body or head. When the defect is inferior it affects mobility because objects below eye level are not visualized. The person with a lower altitudinal defect cannot see the sidewalk, curbs, stairs, or objects directly in the walking path, such as furniture. Inferior defects also make it very difficult to read since usually reading material is held below the central line of sight. The patient may require mobility training and an eccentric viewing pattern. Hemianopic visual field defects are those that are either left or right sided. One half of the peripheral field is either diminished or missing. They render a patient vulnerable to dangers from objects on the blind side. Reading is very difficult when the visual field loss is left-sided because it is hard to find the beginning of the next line of print.

An interesting problem occurs when only a very small island of usable macular vision remains. In this case, patients may experience success with *lower* powers of magnification. Higher powers magnify images right out of the field of view and make reading much more difficult.

When providing low vision aids and making rehabilitation recommendations, the visual field loss should always be taken into account. If a patient does not have a recent visual field in the chart, fields should be assessed as part of the low vision protocol. This does not have to be sophisticated testing. We are not interested in the exact threshold sensitivity of every static point within the field of vision. We are only interested in scotomas or defects that impair function.

An Amsler grid test should be performed on all patients, particularly those with macular degeneration, to look for the location and extent of central scotomas or areas of distortion. Be sure that the patient wears an appropriate reading correction for the distance at which the test is given, and that the central fixation target is marked by a large X or other method so the patient can locate it. A tangent screen is appropriate for those with hemianopic or altitudinal defects. At the very least, a confrontation visual field should be performed to detect gross loss of vision in large areas. A more accurate assessment from a Goldmann or automated perimeter is best. When testing, be sure to take the poor acuity into account. You may need to use a much larger size test object or move the patient closer to the screen to gain an accurate result.

When referring patients for rehabilitation services, include a copy of the visual field with your referral. Visual fields are very helpful in deciding the course of training appropriate for each patient, particularly those with mobility issues.

Step-by-Step Guide to Vision Assessment

1. Measure acuity monocularly with current correction at 10 feet or 5 feet with a test chart that is either handheld or on a movable stand.

2. Record the vision appropriately to reflect the testing distance. (For example, 50-size optotypes seen at a distance of 10 feet would be recorded as 10/50.) Record Snellen equivalents even if using a logMAR chart.

3. Measure near acuity with both eyes open with current lenses and at the currently preferred reading distance.

4. Verify refractive error using a trial frame and full field trial lenses. The vision chart should be at the same distance at which acuity was recorded.

5. Remeasure and record distance acuity monocularly with the new prescription and while the test chart remains at the same distance.

6. After determining the optimal refractive correction, remove a little plus power equivalent to the focal distance of the test chart. (If measured at 10 feet remove 0.25 D, at 5 feet remove between 0.50 and 0.75 D, if closer remove more power accordingly.) This will correct the refractive correction for optical infinity.

7. To begin near testing, place +2.50 lenses over the distance correction still in the trial frame.

8. Hold a near vision reading card at a steady and constant distance of 40 cm and remeasure near reading ability with this combination of lenses. The reading card should have continuous text rather than isolated symbols. Test monocularly. Record the size of type in M units as the denominator and 40 cm as the numerator. For example: The patient reads 4M print at 40 cm; record as 40/4M.

9. Convert the reading ability in M units to a near acuity level. Do this by multiplying 100 times the numerical value (in M units) of the print the patient is able to read. This converts the M number to centimeters. Then divide this centimeter value by 40 to determine the power (in diopters) of the reading add that will most likely allow reading of 1M print. For example: Near vision is 4M.
   4M x 100 = 400 cm
   400 ÷ 40 = 10
   Use a 10 D reading add.

10. Perform contrast sensitivity, visual fields, or other testing as indicated before giving official trials with any aid or making final recommendations.

11. Try the calculated power as a reading add in the trial frame if possible. The same power can be used to try a hand magnifier while the patient looks through his or her distance refractive correction. If a stand magnifier is tried, the magnifier power should be slightly higher and a standard reading add should be used along with it.

Helpful Web Sites

- **Eschenbach Optik of America** (information for professionals)
  www.eschenbach.com/ophthalmologists.php
- **Eye safety and safety glasses information and regulations**
  www.allaboutvision.com/safety
- **Optelec** (for ordering the MN Read cards)
  www.optelec.com or email **Optelec@optelec.com**

References

1. Watson G. Functional assessment of low vision for activities of daily living. In: Silverstone B, Lang MA, Rosenthal B, Faye EE, eds. *The Lighthouse Handbook on Vision Impairment and Vision Rehabilitation.* New York, NY: Oxford University Press; 2000:869-884.

2. Fischer M. Functional evaluation of the adult. In: Silverstone B, Lang MA, Rosenthal B, Faye EE, eds. *The Lightouse Handbook on Vision Impairment and Vision Rehabilitation.* New York, NY: Oxford University Press; 2000:833-853.

3. Sloan LL, Brown DJ. Reading cards for selection of optical aids for the partially sighted. *Am J Ophthalmol.* 1963;55:1187-1199.

Bibliography

Corn A. *Foundations of Low Vision.* New York, NY: American Foundation for the Blind; 1996.

Faye EE, Albert DL, Freed B, Seidman KR, Fischer M. *The Lighthouse Ophthalmology Resident Training Manual: A New Look at Vision Care.* New York, NY: Lighthouse International; 2000.

Holladay J. Guest editorial: visual acuity measurements. *J Cataract Refract Surg.* 2004;30(2):287-290.

Chapter 7

Selecting Aids
for Individuals

KEY POINTS

- Aid selection is determined by the patient's needs and goals as indicated by the history.

- The power of the near aid is determined by the patient's reading ability at a 40 cm testing distance.

- After several trials with a chosen aid, the final determination of whether it is appropriate and affordable will be made by the patient. Follow-up care is always necessary.

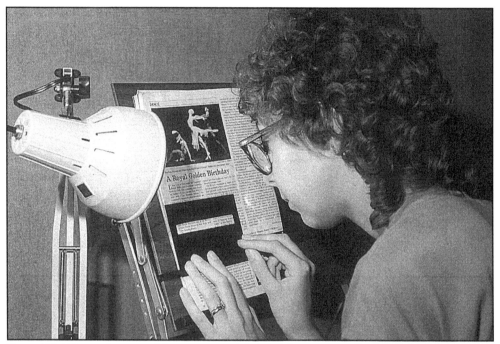

Figure 7-1. When using near vision spectacles it is helpful to use a reading stand to keep the material at a comfortable distance without creating fatigue of the arms. The typoscope helps isolate lines of print and reduces glare.

Among all the available optical and non-optical low vision aids, a specific choice must be made for each patient. Some choices, such as the power and type of optical aid, are made by the primary low vision provider. Other decisions are made mainly by low vision assistants as they work with the patient in follow-up. As patients actually try specific magnifiers, they may decide that a particular model is completely unsatisfactory and a change needs to be made during training. Or it may become evident that a typoscope is necessary to isolate print while using a magnifier (Figure 7-1). For these reasons, low vision assistants should be intimately familiar with the steps to choosing aids and should also keep current with the whole range of non-optical devices and rehabilitation services available.

Deciding on a Style

The first step in choosing an appropriate optical aid is to look at the patient's history. If someone has a task that requires both hands to be free, hand and stand magnifiers are essentially eliminated. Consideration should be limited to spectacles, loupes, and the few freestanding large field magnifiers. You should mentally narrow the choice of magnifiers for each goal of the patient. At the outset, introduce only one or two varieties that solve the most pressing needs of the individual.

For example, consider the case of a woman who loves to knit and do crossword puzzles but also needs to read her mail and recipes. She does not enjoy or desire long-term reading for pleasure. Spectacles, a magnifier on a neckstrap, or a freestanding magnifier would be the best

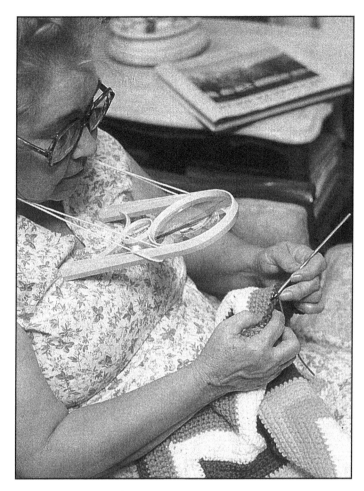

Figure 7-2. A magnifier on a neckstrap keeps the hands free for sewing or crocheting.

choice for her hobbies because they allow freedom of movement for her hands (Figure 7-2). For reading mail, spectacles may be the best option, but a hand or stand magnifier can be considered as well. For reading recipes while cooking, a stand magnifier that sits on the print is best so the vision remains corrected for distance for all other cooking tasks. Spectacles for hobbies, a hand magnifier for mail, and a stand magnifier for reading recipes are good starting choices.

Other case scenarios may indicate consideration of CCTVs and bioptic telemicroscopes. This would be especially true of individuals in college or in visually demanding professions. Severe visual impairment may lead you to suggest voice synthesizers and Braille. Each patient will be very unique.

Determining Power

Conversion of Reading Ability

The second step is to determine the power of magnification necessary for the patient. As discussed in Chapter 6, the method for testing low vision reading acuity is to test the patient's near acuity at a distance of 40 cm with a +2.50 reading add over accurate distance correction and to

Table 7-1
Lens Power/Acuity Chart

Near Acuity Tested at 40 cm

Size of Legible Print	Power of Lens to Try
1M	+2.50
2M	+5.00
3M	+7.50
4M	+10.00
5M	+12.50
7M	+17.50
10M	+25.00

record the smallest size of print that is read fluently. The vision is recorded in the chart as 40 cm over the M units. For example, if the best acuity is 5M, the vision is recorded as 40/5M. Once recorded in this manner, it is easy to put the information into practical use. The patient's reading ability in M units can be converted to dioptric equivalents for each task required.

Think of the notation 40/5M in terms of metric equivalents. The 40 was measured in centimeters, and the 5M refers to 5 meters. Convert the numerator and denominator into like units (centimeters), so now the fraction becomes 40 cm over 500 cm. Divide the denominator by the numerator and it will give you the power of the first lens to try. In this case 500 ÷ 40 = 12.5, so the power of magnifier you will try first is 12.5 D (Table 7-1). (Remember that with stand magnifiers, the power may have to be a bit higher, so start with a 15 D stand magnifier instead of 12.5.)

Providing 12.5 D in spectacles or hand magnifiers should enable this patient to read 1M print. Reading 1M print is considered a useful goal in low vision because it is similar in size to the average typeface in books, magazines, and most professional correspondence. Like the Snellen notation 20/20, however, it is only a standard. A patient may require stronger aids if he or she must read a smaller print size. Another alternative is to use a weaker aid and simply read larger print.

Note: A simpler way to determine power is to use the distance acuity, dividing the denominator by the numerator. For instance, a patient with 20/160 acuity would need an 8 D magnifier. (160 ÷ 20 = 8). This is very simple and can be used in a pinch. Unfortunately, the distance acuity does not always correlate to near reading ability. If you learn to use the 40 cm test above, it will become just as easy to you and will usually be more reliable.

Age of Patient

At this point, the age of the patient is considered. If the patient is phakic and less than 30 years of age, he or she has between 9 D and 16 D of accommodative ability that can supplement the low vision aid power. Always subtract the patient's available accommodative reserve (one half of the total amplitude) from the calculated power requirement before selecting an aid. For example, a 6-year-old patient has 13 D of accommodative ability, so half of that, or 6.5 D, could be used for magnification without fatiguing the eyes. Instead of a 12.5 D magnifier, this child would only need a 6 D lens to read the same material (12.5 - 6.5 = 6). In fact, children often use their entire accommodative ability, holding material close to their eyes in lieu of using any near aid at all. Dividing reserves in half is more practical for those age 12 years and older.

Refractive Error

The patient's refractive error must also be considered when deciding on a power. Patients with myopia have "built-in" plus power and the amount of their refractive error can be subtracted from the power of the aid if it is going to be prescribed in spectacles or used without glasses. A patient with hyperopia needs the calculated power of the aid in addition to the extra plus needed to correct the refractive error. If a patient is going to be wearing glasses or contact lenses that fully correct the refractive error while using a magnifier, the power of the aid remains the same as the calculated power (12.5 D in our example).

Determining Focal Distance

Once appropriate lens power has been determined, calculate the focal distance of that lens. Divide 100 cm by the dioptric power of the lens to get focal length. In our example from the last section, divide 100 by 12.5. The focal length in this case is 8 cm. It is important to note that this focal length does not change if the power of the lens is increased or decreased to incorporate refractive correction of the patient or to allow for accommodation. This focal distance will determine the lens-to-print distance that will be necessary for optimum use of any hand magnifier or reading spectacles. A hand magnifier will be held above the page at a distance equal to the focal distance. Reading material will be held away from the eyes at a distance equal to the focal distance when low vision spectacles are worn.

Visual Field Loss Considerations

When patients have a small scotoma in or near the macula, they usually learn to adapt by looking slightly off-center. This is referred to as eccentric viewing. A patient will turn the eye slightly so the healthy part of the retina is pointing straight ahead to receive the image. Sometimes the position change required for eccentric viewing is very small and the patient will find it easy to adjust. However, patients with a central scotoma larger than 5 degrees in diameter have the most difficulty in reestablishing normal reading patterns. In spite of magnification and a documented improvement in acuity level with low vision aids or refractive correction, these patients always experience a loss of visual efficiency. In one study these patients were only able to read a maximum of 70 words per minute with magnification, while other patients with an intact central visual field but the same acuity level were able to read 130 words per minute.[1]

Sometimes, however, the healthy spot of retina may be further from the fovea or the visual field defect will be very large. In glaucoma, sometimes the entire lower or upper half of the visual field is diminished. Stroke or brain injury may cause a homonymous hemianopia, in which either the entire right or left half of the visual field is missing or diminished.

In some cases the eccentric viewing area causes the patient physical discomfort because of the development of an abnormal head position. Or he or she may experience difficulty in mobility from not being aware of objects in the area of missing visual field. This can sometimes be dealt with successfully by applying Fresnel press-on prisms to the glasses. These prisms move the image of an otherwise unseen object into the area of usable visual field. Sometimes the prisms are placed over one half of the lens to move vision into the half of the usable visual field in patients with homonymous hemianopia. Other times they are applied as a small circle in a particular area only so as to allow the patient awareness of the peripheral visual field when scanning while looking through that portion of the lens. The Gottlieb Visual Field Awareness System™ device developed by Daniel Gottlieb, OD (Stone Mountain, GA), is a similar but permanent attachment to the lenses which holds a clear prism.[2]

Patient Input

Trials in the Office

After an optical low vision aid has been chosen using mathematics and the best experienced opinion of a low vision provider, it still may not be acceptable to the patient. A trial in the office is necessary to help the patient learn to use the aid correctly. In the office, conditions should be ideal. Use a reading stand to hold the book or magazine in place and at the proper angle. Appropriate lighting must be in place, and the reading material should be high contrast 1M-size print. A comfortable chair (without wheels) should be provided so that the only concern of the patient is the use of the optical aid. Instruct your patient on how to hold the lens and where to position it in relation to the eyes and reading material (focal distance). It is important to meet with success at the outset to avoid unnecessary frustration.

Once your patient learns how to use the optical aid he or she should be left to try it alone for a few minutes. Provide ample reading materials including large- and small-print books, newspapers (including the obituary page and crossword puzzle), and typed correspondence (junk mail will do). After this practice session, your patient will either be happy with the lens and willing to try it at home or will have reservations.

The patient's concerns may center on difficulty with field of view or maintaining focal distance. In these cases a little explanation and encouragement will help. However, if the magnification is inadequate or adjustment is very poor, try an alternative low vision aid. While working one-on-one you will become more aware of what the patient desires and how you might improve the situation. You will also discover if the patient is willing to adapt to new situations or is unable to cope with the inherent limitations of magnifiers. This should give you a clue as to how many different aids to try and how much encouragement is needed.

One word of advice: Don't mistake a negative first reaction as failure. This is a new and difficult situation, and not necessarily what this person anticipated when coming for a low vision evaluation. Some people complain a lot, but adapt well to magnifier use with positive encouragement. Don't make rash decisions on changing aids until the patient has had time to try it at home.

Trials at Home

When one or two aids are identified as acceptable under the ideal circumstances you have created in the office, it is time to send the patient home. Keep a stock of aids to lend for home trial, and send most patients home with a magnifier or spectacles in hand on the very first visit. Instruct the patient and an accompanying family member carefully on proper lighting and remind them of the correct focal distance. A written reminder is helpful, because heads are full of new information after an initial low vision exam. It is easiest to keep preprinted pads on hand describing proper lighting and proper use of each major type of aid. Your handout should include several clear and concise steps such as the following, which relate to spectacles.

How to Use Your Low Vision Spectacles

OptT
Optn

- Always maintain a constant distance from your eyes to the paper. For your glasses, this distance is _____ inches.

- A reading stand will help you hold the book at a higher level than your tabletop.

- If the print goes out of focus, bring your face close to the reading material, then back away slowly until the image is clear.

- Always store the glasses in the case provided, as the lenses can become scratched easily. Clean the lenses only with lens cleaner and a soft cloth. Do not rub the lenses with dry paper or cloth.

A similar sheet of instructions can be provided for hand magnifiers, stand magnifiers, and telescopes, as well as lighting. You can be as specific as you wish.

With instructions in hand, patients should be assigned a 1- or 2-week trial in their home or work environment. Actual "homework" assignments should be given to try during the 2 weeks at home. Instruct the patient to try his or her aid in and out of his or her own home with various lighting conditions. Be prepared for some phone calls during this period as patients experience difficulty. Frequently they are unable to function in their home environment as well as they did in the office. Home lighting is worse, and reading stands are probably not available to hold the material at the proper distance. Motivation may also decline as frustration develops and the reality of using the aids daily sinks in.

Follow-Up and Training

The first follow-up visit is generally very productive. Patients are much more able to discuss the advantages and disadvantages of their low vision aid and speak more clearly about specific needs. At this time, power adjustments can be made if print size is still difficult to see. Individuals might tell you spectacles were ideal for home use, but were impossible at the grocery store. A pocket hand magnifier can be recommended.

A woman who plays bridge may complain that spectacles were fine for seeing cards in her own hand, but she was unable to see those on the table. Try half-eye instead of full-frame spectacles so she can look over them, and recommend large-print playing cards. You can also instruct her to ask her partners to say aloud which card is being played.

Another patient may complain that looking up telephone numbers in the directory was difficult. Suggest a small stand magnifier of higher power, placed permanently on the telephone table.

Discuss lighting and reading stands more fully at this time. Also introduce the other non-optical aids that would be most helpful. It is much easier to make suggestions based on very concrete desires. Several such needs will probably be identified at this visit.

What the Patient Needs to Know

- Medicare does not pay for low vision aids. Payment for glasses, magnifiers, and non-optical aids is the patient's responsibility.

- There are agencies who might help you with payment if cost is a prohibitive factor to receiving the aids you need.

- Our office will work with you to try to set up a payment plan or to find alternative methods of payment.

Financial Considerations

Low vision examinations are sometimes covered by insurance, but third-party payers rarely cover the optical aids themselves.

The cost of each low vision aid must be taken into account when recommending it, particularly to patients on fixed incomes. Low power, basic models of optical aids are relatively inexpensive. As of this printing, stock spectacles can range in price from $30 to $200 with increased cost relating to increased power. Frequently these are wholesale prices, so the cost to the patient may be significantly higher. Hand and stand magnifiers range from $3.95 for a simple folding pocket model to $200 or more for lighted stand varieties in attractive designs. The average price for the majority of hand and stand magnifiers is around $40. Low power monocular handheld telescopes cost approximately $20 to $100, while bioptics can run in the $100 to $1,000 range. CCTVs and other electronic devices cost between $1,000 and $4,000.

Be honest with your patients as to the true cost of the devices you recommend. Become familiar with the cost, including your office's markup, so you do not quote the wholesale price from a catalogue to a patient. Cost is one consideration where patient input is mandatory.

Some patients with special circumstances may find agencies that will help meet the financial demands of purchasing optical aids:

- The Veterans Administration will pay for low vision aids for veterans with service-related disabilities.
- Public schools are mandated to provide services to visually impaired students and will usually pay for low vision aids within budget constraints.
- Young adult through middle-aged patients can receive monetary help from state vocational service agencies or services for the blind if the need for low vision aids is vocational in nature.
- The Lions Club civic organization devotes its philanthropic activities to assisting the needs of the blind. Local chapters are often willing to purchase low vision aids for patients who are unable to pay.
- Elder care services, senior centers, and public libraries can be contacted to purchase aids for individuals in the community. These organizations usually purchase a few aids for community use rather than funding individual patients.
- Contact a local civic or school organization to have a "magnifier drive." Older people and their estates frequently donate glasses to the Lions Club, while useful magnifiers are thrown out. If you create a place to donate these items, it could be a good resource for "recycling" aids for use by patients in need.

Step-by-Step Guide to Selecting an Aid

1. Consider the primary goal of the patient. Must the hands be kept free? What is the working distance of each necessary task?

2. Convert the near reading ability from M units to diopters to determine the starting point for trials with optical aids. Remember that the power may be adjusted if the patient's accommodative ability for refractive error warrants it. For instance, a 10 D myope who needs +12 D for reading spectacles will really only need +2 D since the myopia already takes care of 10 D for near. Similarly, if a child needs 12 D for near use and has an accommodative reserve of 12 D, he or she will not need any near correction at all.

3. Determine the focal distance of the chosen magnifier (based on the actual correction, not the adjusted power as described in #2). For instance, the myope will still hold reading material at the focal distance of a +12 D lens even though there is only +2 D in the lenses.

4. Teach the patient to hold the magnifier or reading material at the proper focal distance. Use a reading stand, optimum lighting, and the desired size of printed material.

5. Allow the patient to try it while left alone for a few minutes with other sizes and choices of printed material on hand.

6. Make adjustments in power or style as necessary, considering the patient's financial situation when making decisions.

7. Send the patient home for 1 to 2 weeks to try the selected aid in the home setting. Supply the patient with a trial aid from your loan library as well as preprinted instructions on how to correctly use the aid. If possible, provide the information to a family member as well.

8. On follow-up, listen carefully to the patient's difficulties and successes, making adjustments or recommending additional aids as necessary.

References

1. Higgins KE, Bailey II. Visual disorders and performance of specific tasks requiring vision. In: Silverstone B, Lang MA, Rosenthal B, Faye EE, eds. *The Lighthouse Handbook on Vision Impairment and Vision Rehabilitation.* New York, NY: Oxford University Press; 2000:287-315.

2. Gottlieb DD, Freeman P, Williams M. Clinical research and statistical analysis of a visual field awareness system. *J Am Optom Assoc.* 1992;8:581-588.

Bibliography

Haymes S, Johnston A. Relationship between vision impairment and ability to perform activities of daily living. *Ophthalmic Physiol Opt.* 2002;22(2):79-91.

Chapter 8

The Emotional and Social Aspects of Visual Loss

KEY POINTS

- People who experience loss of vision undergo a grieving period for the "death" of both their previous identity and their independence.

- When partial vision is lost, there is always a fear that total blindness will occur next.

- It is far better for eyecare professionals to be honest than to offer insincere encouragement about prognosis. We should educate and not avoid discussing the realities of visual loss.

Changes in Self-Image

Each time we see a patient who has a disease that leads to loss of vision, we must be aware of what that patient is experiencing at home. We see them when they come to our office, and we hear their answers to the questions we ask when taking the history. Usually the questions we ask are strictly medical: "Has there been any change?" "Have you been looking at your Amsler grid every day?" "Have you noted any new floaters?" The answers to these questions do not give us information about anything in which the patient is interested. Patients are worried that they are going to be totally blind. When we ask if patients have noted any changes, they hear "Has your vision gotten worse like I expect it is going to?" The patient has likely been losing sleep and crying to friends about the fear of blindness. If the vision is poor enough to limit activities of daily living, the patient is also undergoing loss of self-esteem and a multitude of other emotional consequences as a result of the personal adjustments that must be made to adapt to a disability.

In his classic book, *Blindness: What It Is, What It Does, and How to Live With It*,[1] Reverend Thomas J. Carroll outlines 20 substantial losses, or "deaths," of previous characteristics of personal identity that people suffer when they become blind. Some of these losses can also affect the patient with low vision. The magnitude of their impact is related to several factors, including the severity of the visual loss, the age of the patient, concurrent illness or disability, and the level of support from family and friends.[1] Reverend Carroll's list includes many losses that affect different areas of the patient's life, but they can be summarized in the following seven categories discussed below.

Confidence in the Remaining Senses

Many people believe that the remaining senses compensate by becoming sharper when a person is blind. This is not true. In addition, most of the low vision population consists of elderly people. These patients experience the same age-related loss of hearing, taste, and smell as their perfectly sighted contemporaries. Sight is our most reliable sense and is used throughout life to validate the input from the other senses. For instance, when we hear a sound we *glance* in the direction of its origin to verify that it is, in fact, the sound we thought. Without the ability to validate the other senses by visual verification, low vision patients become afraid of their own ability to make sensory judgments. Vision has always been automatically used as a "double check" to sensory inputs from taste, smell, and touch as well. Now the person must completely reorient him- or herself to other environmental clues. It is this reorienting of attention paid to the other senses that makes them seem as if they are more acute. Actually it is just the *focus* on them that is now stronger.

Orientation and Mobility

Orientation refers to our ability to know where we are in the environment at any given time. This might be finding a room in the house, locating a particular street address or a desired office in a large building, or even literally knowing the way out of the woods. *Mobility* refers to our ability to move about independently in that environment and reach the destination we seek. When vision decreases, this independence is compromised in many ways. When a driver's license is denied, the world quickly becomes a smaller place. It also creates a dependence that many find very difficult to accept. Suddenly it is necessary to ask for help with menial trips, such as running to the bank or post office, and with more important ones like getting to work or medical appointments.

Even if public transportation is available, people with low vision often avoid its use for safety reasons. They fear they might fall down stairs, read the wrong signs on the bus or subway, get off at the wrong stop, or become stranded from inability to read a timetable or clock. Even walking can be difficult when one cannot see the traffic signals at street corners or from the fear of tripping over stones or loose pavement. Often a loss of vision causes people to stay home, and then they become isolated and susceptible to depression.

Daily Living Tasks

When vision is poor it becomes very difficult to tell if your home or clothes are dirty or soiled, which can lead to unwitting negligence of cleaning or grooming. This is frustrating for the person who has always taken pride in his or her appearance and surroundings. Not only is it difficult to tell if there is a problem with dust or dirt, but it is challenging to carry out the tasks necessary to remedy it. Shaving, applying makeup, and other grooming tasks also become chores.

Cooking is difficult when vision is not sufficient to read measuring cups or to set timers and temperatures. Shopping is difficult when you have a lack of transportation and then experience difficulty reading prices or seeing well enough to write a check.

Communication

When vision loss affects the size of print that can be read easily, it becomes difficult to read one's own mail, correspond with friends and businesses, and enjoy the daily paper. Although this particular challenge is widely recognized and can usually be improved with the use of magnifiers, it should not be the only issue that is addressed during a low vision examination. Other types of communication that can be disrupted from decreased vision include computer use, email or instant messaging, and the ability to look up phone numbers. Using a cellular phone becomes difficult, especially as the models become smaller and have more information on a tiny screen.

Communication also becomes difficult when speaking face to face with another person. In conversations we do more than hear the words of others. We watch their facial expressions and gestures for clues as to the humor or actual intentions of the words. Frequently we can tell more about a person from the look on his or her face than from the words that are spoken. Those unable to see the speaker are at the mercy of the words alone, leading to awkwardness in many social situations. Another aspect of this problem is being unable to recognize friends when passing them on the street or at social gatherings. A person who loses sight may now be perceived as being unfriendly by unwitting acquaintances. This is especially true for low vision patients who are able to function fairly normally and show no outward signs of their disability. Many relationships suffer as a result of this misunderstanding.

Financial Security and Career or Vocational Goals

The loss of a job is a major issue for adults below retirement age. When the ability to function in a job is gone we not only lose our income, but also the identity that we have fashioned for ourselves over many years of working. This identity can no longer be lived up to, and the financial security the job provided can be compromised. For younger adults, their dreams of the future with a particular career can be dashed. They may be forced to consider a new job option that is less interesting and less financially lucrative. They might fear that their future life will be less appealing or fulfilling.

This loss of satisfying employment and income due to low vision frequently occurs at the same time that expenses increase. There are more doctor and pharmacy bills, more fees for transportation to appointments, and perhaps less insurance coverage. Because of the decrease in ability to perform tasks of daily living, there may also be expenses from hiring delivery people, housekeepers, and visiting helpers to read mail or perform other tasks.

Another problem with finances occurs from an inability to read bills, write checks, or fill out tax forms. Often low vision patients, particularly elderly ones, become less timely in the paying of bills and can become stressed by overdue notices and charges. When recommending low vision aids, be sure to consider the cost of the particular aids in the context of the financial hardship a patient may be experiencing. A person with little income may not be able to afford an electronic reading machine even if it is proven to be the best type of aid for improving his or her reading ability.

Personal Independence and Self-Esteem

When a person's vision fails, it becomes difficult to be at peace with the identity of "self" that has been developed over a lifetime. Suddenly the person thinks of him- or herself as disabled, and for many people that carries negative connotations beyond the life changes that occur. There may be guilt over some profession or habit that he or she thinks caused his or her eyes to go bad, or feel that the situation is the payback for some sin that he or she committed. There is often a fear of imminent total blindness as well. People in the community can exacerbate the feeling by expressing pity for the person and beginning to treat him or her differently. This change can be interpreted by the disabled person as being stigmatized, and lead to a feeling of social separation.

One of the worst causes of depression that follows visual loss is from the patient's lack of independence and control over his or her own life. Sometimes family members and friends mean well in their efforts, but increase the patient's dependence by helping too much. These caregivers take over the performance of regular tasks, rather than helping their family member return to a state of independence. As Reverend Carroll so aptly states, "Death to independence means an end to adult living."[1]

Recreation and Personal Enjoyment

Recreation includes anything done for pleasure, such as sports, games, needlework, movie-going, or collecting. Many activities previously engaged in for sheer enjoyment become difficult or impossible. Also, as vision decreases people are no longer able to accurately see the faces of their loved ones, appreciate their own jewelry, enjoy looking at the details in artwork, or derive satisfaction from any of the many ways we delight in life through looking at lovely things.

Recreation and sports provide outlets for stress as well. When customary recreational activities must be abandoned, part of the normal ability to decrease stress is lost as well. Since one of the major results of compromised vision is an increase in stress, the need for an outlet is even more important. So when it becomes difficult to continue recreation and physical activities, stress levels rise even further.

Many, if not all, of these difficulties occur in each individual we see as low vision patients, even though they are manifested in differing ways and differing intensities. When the visual decline occurs slowly over a long period of time, these problems may take a long time to work through. Some patients try so desperately to rely on their vision that they do not realize when it is time to relearn ways of doing things.

For instance, sometimes as a visual field begins to deteriorate from glaucoma the patient does not really notice the loss. Without realizing it, the person might develop a compensating head turn to see things that are further in the periphery. However, as the field continues to worsen, this adaptive head position can become a hindrance rather than a help. When crossing streets, for example, the need to see the white line and look for curbs causes the person to be bent over and unaware of anything else in the area. This persistent reliance on visual clues rather than trusting of other senses can render the person unable to walk alone. A mobility aid such as a long cane or dog would go a long way to help this person stand upright and use the remaining vision more efficiently (eg, to look at the walk/don't walk sign or the traffic light rather than the ground). But since the visual field loss is so gradual, it may take a long time before this patient is able to come around to this new way of doing things. It usually takes an orientation and mobility instructor to teach these new techniques and help the person regain independence.

What the Patient Needs to Know

- Adjusting to visual loss requires mourning the loss of your independence. It is normal to be sad, frightened, and depressed.

- There are other people experiencing the same difficulties as you. We can put you in touch with others who are sharing your same fears if you would like some peer support.

- There is hope. Other people have achieved great things in spite of total blindness. Although you will not be able to function as you did before, you can still function at a very high level.

For other patients, if the visual loss is more sudden, the problems of dealing with it can be much more acute and result in near paralysis of ability to function for a while. Most low vision patients go through stages of acceptance similar to the stages of grief. These might include shock, disbelief, anger, mourning, depression, and finally coping skills and the return of self-esteem. These stages do not necessarily occur in order, nor do they occur at the same intensity or for the same length of time in all patients.

Some of the factors that influence a person's ability to move smoothly to the stage of acceptance and the return of self-esteem include the presence of other health concerns, level of social isolation, and the length of time since the onset of visual loss. Diabetic patients, whose vision fluctuates and remains unstable, have a harder time coping than do patients with a stable vision loss. This is true even if the stable visual acuity is worse than the fluctuating loss.

Age is also a factor in adjustment. Patients under the age of 15 and those over the age of 51 have been found to cope fairly well, while those aged 16 to 50 experience more anger and depression from their vision loss.[2]

Taking all of these factors into consideration, it becomes clear that a patient may not be receptive to low vision aids until he or she has had the time to work through the emotional adjustments. It is only with full acceptance that a patient will let go of old habits and relearn new ways of doing things and new adaptive techniques. This comes easily to some, with difficulty to others, and to still others it is never possible. We must understand when we suggest low vision aids that the patient who is unsuccessful just may be unable to accept the necessity of the visual aid. Given time, that same person may be willing to admit that his or her vision is not going to improve, but probably will not decline further either. Only at that time will an aid be accepted. The same patient who was unsuccessful originally may be the most successful once the visual loss has been accepted.

Reactions of Families and Friends

The support of family and friends is another very important factor in the ability of a patient to cope with low vision. Generally families are anxious to help their relative achieve independence, and sometimes are concerned about it earlier than is the patient him- or herself. Sometimes a patient is more anxious about the treatment than a return to independence, and the encouragement of family members is helpful along the road to adjustment. A supportive family environment allows the patient to regain a sense of self-control and self-esteem that those in isolation do not experience. However, even in the absence of strong family support, patients can do well with the help of a group of friends or caring professionals. When a patient feels that someone still believes in him or her, and also encourages a return to independence, the person moves more quickly toward accepting the disability.

There are also families that hinder the adjustment process rather than help it. Some families have a hard time accepting the vision loss and so are not as supportive as they need to be. Problems usually fall into two camps. First are the families who overreact and want to take care of the patient. These families are easy to spot. They always fuss over the patient as he or she walks into the room. They hold on to him or her until safely seated in the chair, jump up at any sign of need, and frequently speak for the patient as well. These families mean well, but can be a great hindrance to the patient's ability to regain his or her self-esteem, self-worth, and independence. If someone is taking care of all your needs, it is impossible to take responsibility for yourself.

What the Patient Needs to Know

- You are not stupid, you are only disabled.

- Other people will not understand your disability unless you inform them. They do not mean to be insensitive, they simply do not understand.

The second difficult type of family is one steeped in denial. Low vision patients almost always look normal. They do not have any outward signs of their handicap, and nothing external has changed. Except for patients with debilitating visual field loss, patients can usually walk alone and take care of most of their own responsibilities. The family does not understand (and often does not believe) when Mother cannot shop alone or keep up with correspondence. The family members believe that she is just looking for sympathy or acting lazy when she asks for help or complains about her inability to function. This type of family can be very devastating, causing the patient to pretend to be much more self-sufficient than he or she really is. Long-term problems can result, such as mistakes in paying bills, accidents while cooking or attempting to drive, and the emotional inability to ask for help when it is needed.

This lack of awareness of visual loss is also manifested by friends and acquaintances. A low vision person can be perceived by friends as being suddenly clumsy or stupid. Others may doubt the visually impaired person's intelligence when they consistently play the wrong card or write down the wrong phone number. They are perceived as being unfriendly when in fact they cannot see the faces of people across the room. All of these misunderstandings can lead anyone to begin to decline social invitations, leading to loneliness and depression. Each of these problems can be exacerbated if the patient lets pride get in the way and does not explain to peers that he or she is experiencing a visual loss.

Reactions of Health Professionals

`OphA`
`OphMT`
`OptA`
`OptT`

As health professionals we are also guilty of avoidance and denial. Often when dealing with low vision patients we tell them how well they are doing. We praise them for reading the 20/100 line this visit when last week they were only able to read 20/100-1. It is easy to say, "Oh, your vision is much better this time." Although innocently meant as encouragement, this type of behavior helps lead the patients to denial and false hope. They look to their eye appointments with great anticipation, and the comments of eyecare professionals become very important. If we tell patients they are doing better, they think they hear that their vision is going to improve and they are going to "get better." This type of false hope only leads to a delay in the patient's ability to accept the visual loss and seek help in dealing with it. This in turn stands in the way of regaining self-esteem and independence.

What the Patient Needs to Know

- Using your eyes will not harm them. Nothing you did in the past has caused you to lose your vision.

- Low vision is a term that means that your vision is poor. It does not mean that you are blind or that you will become blind.

- We in eyecare want to do everything we can to enable you to see well. Sometimes we can no longer make your vision better. But we can help you adjust to your new situation if you will work with us.

- If you misunderstand the meaning of your eye disease or are not sure what it means for your future, please ask. Although we understand your fears in general, we are not aware of specific concerns until you mention them.

What You Can Do to Help

Honesty and Tact

`OphMT`

When dealing with patients who are experiencing visual loss, realize that addressing the difficulties is not going to embarrass them. It may disappoint them, but honesty is always best. Eyecare professionals should talk to patients honestly and without pity or condescension. First and foremost, the diagnosis must be explained fully in laymen's terms. If the patient does not understand what is wrong with his or her eyes, fear and misunderstanding will result. The prognosis should be completely explained as well. If the vision is going to remain poor, it should be recognized as such. False encouragement should not be given. If the vision is 20/100 for several months, it is far better to let the patient know that you understand he or she must be experiencing difficulties in daily life. Ask what types of problems he or she is encountering and suggest some non-optical aids that might help. This would also be a good time to offer a copy of a non-optical aids catalogue, even before a formal low vision evaluation. During this explanation of visual loss, all patients must be reassured that the loss of vision is not due to any action on their own part. Most patients fear that they have done something in the past to harm their eyes such as read too much, sew too much, or watch television in the dark. Reassure each patient that using their eyes will not harm them. Otherwise, they might stop attempting to read or function visually.

Since family support is imperative to adjustment, it is important to include the family members in any discussion with the patient. However, do not talk to the family members and ignore the patient. Always address the patient directly, asking your questions to him or her and not to family members. If a caretaker tries to answer for the patient, tactfully ask that the patient be allowed to answer. Caretakers do have important information, so listen to what they have to say as well, but only after informing the patient you are going to do so. By your example, caretakers will learn to allow the patient autonomy and independence. The patient will learn that you value his or her opinion and judgment and will be more likely to open up about needs and concerns. If clinicians talk mainly to family members, it gives the patient the impression of being devalued and will cause a level of distrust which will hinder progress in the low vision evaluation.

Use the terminology the patient will need in the future. Discuss the idea of "low vision," and how it is different than blindness. Let the patient know that while vision is poor, it is not going to be completely lost. Also be honest that he or she is probably not going to note much improvement, either. Many patients are confused about the term "legal blindness." Educate each patient on the difference between low vision, legal blindness, and total blindness. Mention the existence of low vision services, and offer a referral when they feel ready. All of this can be done while the patient still considers laser and other treatments.

Our own attitudes toward blindness and rehabilitation color our treatment of patients with poor vision. If we are afraid of blindness, we will be afraid to be encouraging. If we feel that rehabilitation is some type of nightmare to be avoided, we will not refer our patients properly. If we feel that blindness is a failure in the eyecare system, we will feel disillusioned and attempt to avoid dealing with the consequences.

The best way to overcome these false ideas is to visit a rehabilitation center for the blind. When eyecare professionals are educated in the possibilities open to partially sighted individuals they will feel more comfortable and make appropriate referrals. A visit to a local center for the blind is recommended for every person in eyecare, but most particularly to those who are setting up a low vision service.

Patients with severe loss of vision may not recognize who you are, or even when you enter or leave the room. If a patient cannot see your face, he or she is not sure if you are speaking to him or her or to someone else in the room. Always say the patient's name when addressing him or her, and introduce yourself in the same context. Physical contact, such as a touch of the shoulder or handshake, are also reassuring and help the person know your proximity. This can be simply done as you call the patient in from the waiting room. "Hi Mr. Davis, I'm Linda, the low vision assistant. I'll walk with you to the exam room and we'll see how you are doing with your new glasses."

Support Groups

Loss of vision is very isolating, and each patient who experiences it feels alone and frightened. The ability to share the experience with others who are experiencing a similar loss is invaluable. You or your office can offer an extremely valuable service to your patients by facilitating a way for patients to meet. There are several ways this can be accomplished depending on the interest and enthusiasm of your office staff:

- A bimonthly evening session can be offered in your office or at a local meeting hall. If desired, it can be solely a social gathering, with your office merely coordinating the place to meet and sending out flyers to the appropriate patients.
- The sessions can be more formal, with a guest speaker and social hour each time. Guest speakers can be invited from local rehabilitation agencies, low vision aid vendors, low vision clinics, and other support or informational groups.
- Alternatively, patients from your office can be given the names and phone numbers of other consenting patients so they can call one another with questions or support.
- Patients with similar diagnoses and poor vision can be scheduled for their follow-up eye appointments on the same afternoon each month. Then the lunch hour can be set aside for them to meet one another if they want to come early to the appointment. (Many patients who need help with transportation come to visits early anyway.) This way, there would be something positive for them to do while they are waiting. One day per month could be "macular degeneration day," one day could be "diabetic retinopathy day," etc. That way the patients do not have to go to another site to make contact with one another.

Other ways of putting patients in contact with one another are as numerous as your imagination will allow. Providing patients with the opportunity to share experiences can only be helpful and ease them through their transition into a mentally healthy low vision person ready for low vision aids and rehabilitation. It is important, however, to try to arrange for patients in different stages of adjustment to attend these meetings. If all the patients have been recently diagnosed, they may only share their fears and resentments. People who have worked through their loss, adjusted to visual aids, and once again gained independence are important role models. They should be available to offer encouragement and hope for the future.

Although children adapt very well to vision loss, parents of these children are devastated and afraid. They are usually very receptive to the idea of meeting other parents in a similar situation and appreciative of information about support groups. You can form one of these groups, encourage parents of your visually impaired pediatric patients to form them, or direct the parents to a group sponsored by established organizations. Local chapters of the National Association for Parents of Children with Visual Impairments (NAPVI) are available around the country. By contacting the national branch in Watertown, MA, parents can get information and support from other parents. The address for NAPVI is given in Chapter 9 (see page 117).

Helpful Web Sites

Support Organizations About Children
- National Association for Parents of Children with Visual Impairments
  www.spedex.com/napvi
- National Organization of Parents of Blind Children
  www.nfb.org/nopbc/

Support and Advocacy Organizations for Adults
- American Council of the Blind
  www.acb.org
- American Foundation for the Blind
  www.afb.org
- Council of Citizens with Low Vision International
  www.cclvi.org
- National Association for Visually Handicapped
  www.navh.org
- National Federation of the Blind
  www.nfb.org

Specific Diagnoses and Their Support Networks
- Albinism
  www.albinism.org
- Diabetes
  www.diabetes.org
- Glaucoma
  www.wills-glaucoma.org/support.htm
- Macular degeneration
  www.mdsupport.org/
- Retinitis pigmentosa
  www.rpinternational.org
- Others: Contact **www.lowvision.org/disease** for a list of many other diagnoses and their support networks

Patient-Friendly General Information Sites
- E-medicine
  www.emedicine.com/oph
- Low Vision Center
  www.lowvisioninfo.org
- NIH Information for Elderly Patients
  http://nihseniorhealth.gov/lowvision/toc.html
- OcuSource (find doctors, therapists, manufacturers, and organizations for the blind and partially sighted)
  www.ocusource.com

References

1. Carroll T. *Blindness: What It Is, What It Does, and How to Live With It.* Boston, MA: Little, Brown & Co; 1961.

2. Ringering L, Amaral P. The role of psychosocial factors in adaptation to vision impairment and rehabilitation outcomes for adults and older adults. In: Silverstone B, Lang MA, Rosenthal B, Faye EE, eds. *The Lighthouse Handbook on Vision Impairment and Vision Rehabilitation.* New York, NY: Oxford University Press; 2000:1029-1045.

Bibliography

Dickman I. *What Can We Do About Limited Vision?* New York, NY: Public Affairs Pamphlet; 1977.

Emerson D. Facing loss of vision: the responses of adults to visual impairment. *The Journal of Visual Impairment and Blindness.* 1981;2:41-45.

Horowitz A, Silverstone B, Reinhardt J. A conceptual and empirical exploration of personal autonomy issues within family caregiving relationships. *Gerontologist.* 1991;31(1):23-31.

Stotland J. Relationship of parents to professionals: a challenge to professionals. *The Journal of Visual Impairment and Blindness.* 1984;2:69-74.

Chapter 9

Rehabilitation and Referrals

KEY POINTS

- State-run and private agencies are available to help your patients. Check with your state government for local details.

- Professionals who provide assistance to blind or low vision patients include: vision rehabilitation therapists, rehabilitation counselors, teachers of the visually impaired, orientation and mobility specialists, and occupational therapists.

Agencies and Professionals Who
Help People Adjust to Vision Loss

Agencies for the blind have been operating in the United States for generations. Blindness was one of the first disabilities to be recognized and adopted by philanthropic organizations. Because of this there are hundreds of agencies, organizations, and self-help and advocacy groups available to your patients. The following is a general overview to make you aware of the various types of organizations available. A brief synopsis of the professionals who work with visually impaired patients is also provided.

Federal Government Services

People who meet federal criteria for legal blindness have many services and financial benefits available to them.

The Social Security Administration offers two possibilities, Social Security Disability Insurance (SSDI) and Supplemental Security Income (SSI). SSDI is available to people who have paid into the Social Security retirement system. After a 5-month waiting period, they are eligible for a monthly financial disability compensation. They will also be referred to a vocational rehabilitation counselor for retraining in the same career or a new one so they can remain self-sufficient and productive. SSI is another monetary benefit available to anyone who is disabled or age 65 or older if financial need is demonstrated. It is a monthly payment to help with the costs of daily living. Social Security's web site is www.ssa.gov/pubs/10052.html. They have a useful publication entitled *How We Can Help* which describes benefits for blind and visually impaired people.

The US Postal Service offers postage-free mailing to the blind and visually impaired. This rate can be used to send any recorded or large-print items. The Internal Revenue Service offers a deduction for blindness on federal tax forms.

All of these benefits and more are offered to patients once they are referred to a state agency for the blind. Be sure to refer your patients as soon as possible, so they are aware of all possible services. Even if they do not meet the criteria for legal blindness, low vision patients may be eligible for some of these services depending on their level of disability.

State Agencies

All states have an office that oversees support of blind and low vision individuals. Sometimes it is a separate agency specifically devoted to blindness, such as the Commission for the Blind in Massachusetts. Sometimes it is a division of another agency, such as education; vocational services; or health, education, and welfare. Sometimes the support is splintered between several agencies. For instance, the department of education may handle children, vocational services may handle adults, and welfare may handle senior citizens, each within a separate subdivision of blind services. However they are organized, these agencies coordinate rehabilitation centers, public school assistance, and residential schools for the blind. They also provide monetary and vocational support to blind individuals.

Most states offer services to low vision individuals as well as to their totally blind clients, but often have some restriction based on acuity level and age. Some people may only be able to receive services if their vision loss falls into the category of legal blindness. Exceptions are usually made for those who have a poor prognosis, for children in public schools, or for those whose disability results in a loss of vocation. Services offered vary widely from state to state, so contact your state government for details. To find contact information for your state, go to the National Council of State Agencies for the Blind web site: www.ncsab.org/ncsab_directory.htm.

Advocacy and Support Groups

There is a support group for almost all visual impairments and concerns. Specifically for children, the Hadley School offers free courses by home study on issues related to parents and children with visual impairments.

Hadley School for the Blind
700 Elm St
Winnetka, IL 60093
800-323-4238

The National Association for Parents of Children with Visual Impairments (NAPVI) is a national organization for parents with visually impaired children. They have an information exchange for parents and can put parents of children with similar disabilities in contact with one another. They publish a quarterly newsletter called *Awareness* that updates parents on social, medical, and educational resources for their children. It also provides information on pertinent legislation, conferences, and activities. In addition, NAPVI is a clearinghouse regarding support services for rare eye disorders, parenting issues, and information on government agencies of help to families with a blind or low vision child.

National Association for Parents of Children with Visual Impairments
PO Box 317
Watertown, MA 02471
Local chapters have individual phone numbers. See the web site for details:
www.spedex.com/napvi

Similar groups for adults, which also engage in lobbying for blindness issues, are the National Federation of the Blind (NFB) and the American Council of the Blind (ACB). In addition, both organizations sponsor special interest affiliate groups. The ACB sponsors the Visually Impaired Veterans of America as well as the Library Users of America, and publishes the *Braille Forum*, a free monthly magazine with information pertinent to blindness issues. The NFB sponsors the National Organization of Parents of Blind Children and also offers a free talking newspaper service (available on a toll-free phone number) called *NFB-Newsline*. Members can call and hear the complete text of many daily newspapers nationwide.

American Council of the Blind
1155 15th St NW, Suite 1004
Washington, DC 20005
800-424-8666
www.acb.org

National Federation of the Blind
1800 Johnson St
Baltimore, MD 21230
410-659-9314
Local affiliates have local phone numbers. See information on the web site: www.nfb.org.

The Council of Citizens with Low Vision International (CCLVI) and the National Association for Visually Handicapped (NAVH) provide information and advocacy specifically to low vision individuals (vs the totally blind). NAVH provides public and professional education, sells low vision aids, and houses a 9,000-volume lending library of large-print books that can be borrowed free by mail. CCLVI provides public and professional education, advocates legislation that helps people with low vision, and provides outreach to ensure that people are getting the services they require.

Council of Citizens with Low Vision International
906 N Chambliss St
Alexandria, VA 22312
800-733-2258
www.cclvi.org

National Association for Visually Handicapped
22 W 21st St, 6th Floor
New York, NY 10010
212-255-2804
      or
507 Polk St, Suite 420
San Francisco, CA 94102
415-775-6284
www.navh.org

The American Foundation for the Blind offers a multitude of services and information to blind and low vision individuals as well as low vision providers. They provide information on most topics and publish pamphlets, books, and journals related to blindness issues. They also can be contacted for information on referrals and state regulations nationwide. Lighthouse International offers low vision training to professionals and provides medical and rehabilitation services to blind and low vision clients.

American Foundation for the Blind
11 Penn Plaza, Suite 300
New York, NY 10001
800-232-5463
www.afb.org

Lighthouse International Headquarters
The Sol and Lillian Goldman Bldg
111 E 59th St
New York, NY 10022
212-821-9200
www.lighthouse.org

The National Library Service for the Blind and Physically Handicapped (NLS) is a free national library program originating in the Library of Congress. They provide recorded and Braille versions of 423,000 full-length books and 70 periodicals. There is also a music section which provides large-print and Braille music scores and textbooks, as well as cassette recordings of lectures and musical instruction. These reading materials are distributed free of charge through regional and local libraries to people who are eligible due to visual or physical impairment. The reading matter and the playback machines are borrowed and returned through the US Mail with a special postage-free rate for the blind and visually impaired. They can also be accessed on the Internet through Web-Braille. The NLS (see page 41 for address) has a special application form that includes a section to be completed by an ophthalmologist or optometrist. Copies of this application should be on hand in your office.

People who work with blind individuals may join the Association for Education and Rehabilitation of the Blind and Visually Impaired (AER). Visually impaired workers themselves can belong to organizations such as the National Association of Blind Teachers, the American Blind Lawyers Association, or the Visually Impaired Information Specialists, Inc.

Association for Education and Rehabilitation of the Blind and Visually Impaired
1703 N Beauregard St, Suite 440
Alexandria, VA 22311
877-492-2708
www.aerbvi.org

There are recreational groups, such as Blind Outdoor Leisure Development (BOLD Inc, Aspen, Colo, www.challengeaspen.com/Recreation/bold) and Ski for Light (Minneapolis, Minn, www.sfl.org), that coordinate camping and skiing trips for visually impaired children and adults. There is a blind golfer's association (www.blindgolf.com) and several groups sponsored by the ACB, such as the Blind Radio Amateurs and Friends-in-Art for poorly sighted artists and art lovers (www.acb.org/affiliates).

Support groups for various conditions include the Helen Keller Services for the Blind (www.helenkeller.org), the Retinitis Pigmentosa Foundation (www.rpinternational.org), the National Organization for Albinism and Hypopigmentation (www.albinism.org), and the American Diabetes Association (www.diabetes.org).

What the Patient Needs to Know

- Vision rehabilitation therapists will teach you methods to perform tasks of daily living.

- Rehabilitation counselors can provide you with options for vocational training and advise you on where to receive help.

- Teachers of the visually impaired work closely with children in public schools to make sure their educational and rehabilitation needs are being met.

- Orientation and mobility specialists will teach you to travel independently in your home or in public places.

- Occupational therapists working in clinics can teach you to use low vision aids or other appliances efficiently and to perform other tasks of daily living.

Rehabilitation Personnel

Rehabilitation Counselors

Rehabilitation counselors are professionals who provide vocational assistance and information to blind and low vision clients. They develop and maintain files on each individual in their caseload and coordinate services provided by various organizations. Primarily hired by state agencies or rehabilitation centers, these individuals are similar to school counselors. They provide information and referrals. They may also act as social workers, dealing with the adjustment and concerns of the blind client and family members. They frequently advocate for their clients in obtaining services from educational or vocational institutions. They also coordinate monetary support from federal agencies to fund the needs of clients. Rehabilitation counselors are a good contact for low vision clinics, as they are usually aware of the resources available for each patient.

Vision Rehabilitation Therapists

Vision rehabilitation therapists (VRTs), formerly known as rehabilitation teachers, are more specific therapists. They work in rehabilitation centers, residential schools for the blind, and large public schools. They may also work on an itinerant basis traveling to public schools in less populated areas, to the workplace, or to the client's home to provide individual instruction.

Activities of VRTs may include helping an elderly person organize kitchen cabinets by labeling each shelf front with a Braille or large-print sticker. They may teach Braille. They work with low vision patients in their homes, helping with the use of a magnifier or providing non-optical aids. They help arrange the workplace in a useful manner for easier use by someone with low vision (Figure 9-1). VRTs work in a very hands-on manner and are a helpful resource for low vision clinics, as they can provide follow-up training after patients leave your office. If you are fortunate enough to work closely with a VRT, you can provide detailed instructions that can be invaluable to your patient's success with low vision aids.

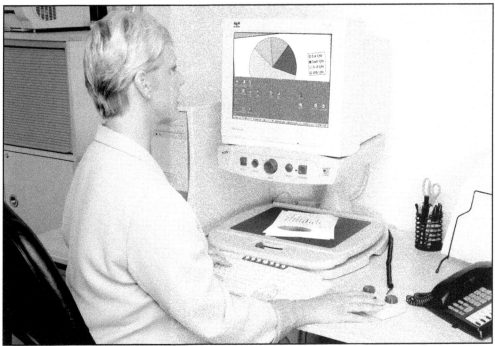

Figure 9-1. Many clients of vision rehabilitation therapists learn to use all computer skills so they can remain employed. (Photo courtesy of Enhanced Vision, Huntington Beach, CA.)

Orientation and Mobility Instructors (Peripatologists)

Orientation and mobility (O&M) instructors are the professionals responsible for teaching clients to move around in their environment in spite of limited vision. They work in residential centers, rehabilitation centers, and schools on a full-time or itinerant basis.

O&M instructors teach clients to become oriented to their surroundings by paying attention to sounds, landmarks, and clues. They teach clients to maneuver in their home setting by using self-protective techniques and arranging furniture and supplies in an organized manner. Orientation to the school or workplace is provided, and they also explain the logical arrangement of address numbering systems and street grids, enabling clients to use public transportation and find their own way in any private or public environment.

Long Cane Travel

The use of a long cane, otherwise known as a white cane, is taught by O&M instructors during the course of mobility training (Figure 9-2). These canes work as an extension of the person's arm and provide tactile feedback about the environment that is about to be traversed. Canes are excellent tools for detecting curbs, walkways, barriers, and changes in terrain. They cannot, however, warn their user of obstacles or dangers outside an approximately 3-foot radius in front of them. Most long cane users rely on them to provide confidence that they are walking in the correct direction and on a safe walking surface. They also give subtle clues about when a curb is approaching, a driveway is being crossed, and other information that assists in reacting safely to the environment.

Figure 9-2. An orientation and mobility instructor teaches long cane travel.

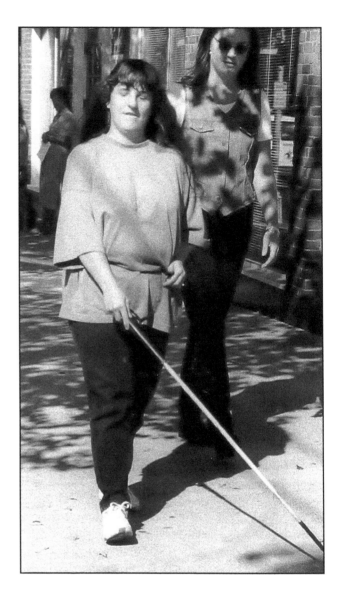

Guide Dogs

Guide dogs are another form of mobility "device" that function much like a long cane. These dogs are trained to warn their master of any object in, or heading toward, their path that should be avoided (Figure 9-3). Besides the fact that they can be great companions, dogs are better than canes in several ways. A guide dog that is "working" will continually scan the area for danger. It looks out for walking hazards, such as potholes, curbs, stairs, and downed limbs, or obstacles that might strike its master's head, as well as for cars or bicycle riders and other dangers such as threatening animals or would-be muggers.

Guide dogs are not for every individual, however. The blind person must be in good physical condition. The master must be fast enough to keep up with the pace of a healthy dog, and strong enough to control the animal. Guide dogs can become lazy if they do not work daily, so the person who uses one must have a daily routine that takes them both out walking. Reevaluation and retraining of dogs is necessary from time to time. (Note: It is incorrect to refer to guide dogs

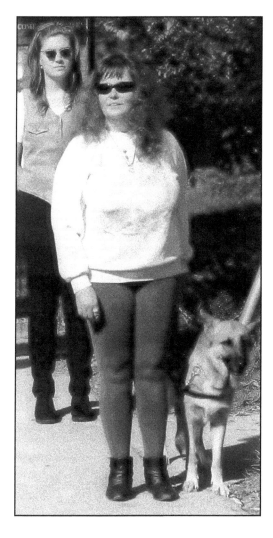

Figure 9-3. A guide dog is aware of dangers that a cane cannot detect and is an excellent companion. Orientation and mobility training is necessary with a dog as well as a cane.

as "seeing eye dogs." The Seeing Eye is one guide dog center in New Jersey that is very well known. There are, however, many other centers that provide excellent guide dogs for the blind. The appropriate term to use is "guide dog.")

Sighted Guide Training

OphA

O&M instructors also teach clients a technique known as "sighted-guide travel." This is when a blind or partially sighted individual holds onto the arm of a sighted person who guides him or her in unfamiliar surroundings. There will be many instances when a low vision provider will have to function as a sighted guide in the office, clinic, or hospital, so some of the rules are important to know.

- When guiding a blind person, always make contact first by touching the back of his or her hand with the back of yours, and stating that you will be happy to guide him or her to your destination (Figure 9-4). This allows the person to locate you and place his or her hand in the correct position on your arm. He or she will grasp your arm from behind and slightly above the elbow (Figure 9-5). You can offer more support to elderly or unsure individuals if necessary by allowing them to lean on your bent arm. (If your

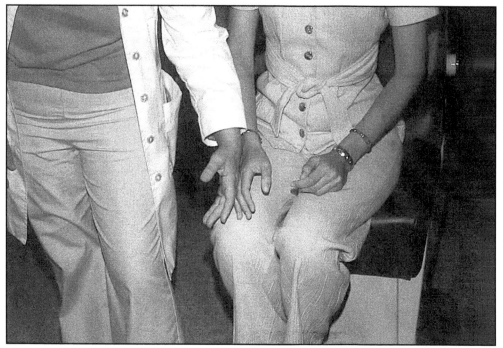

Figure 9-4. Touch the back of your hand to the back of the patient's hand. This provides the patient the option of taking your arm or walking independently.

contact is rejected, allow the patient to walk on his or her own. Some people do not like to be guided.)

- Always allow the person to hold your arm and walk a half pace behind you. Never guide him or her in front of you. You must walk ahead and be the leader, thereby giving clues through your body movements as to when to start, stop, slow down, or turn.

- If you must step up or down stairs, stop completely on the landing and tell the person you are guiding that there are stairs. Allow him or her to hold the handrail with his or her free hand, maintaining contact with your arm. Begin to ascend or descend the stairs at a slow but regular pace. Do not pause until you reach the end of the staircase, but stop fully on the final landing to let the person know that you have reached the end. Allow them to catch up to you completely before proceeding.

- If you come to a doorway, open the door yourself, but allow the person you are guiding to close it behind you.

- When seating the person you are guiding, stop fully and remove his or her hand from your arm. Place that hand on the seat of the chair, and explain that he or she should sit down. If there is a footrest in the way, either remove it or explain that it is there.

If you follow these basic sighted-guide procedures, your patients will feel more comfortable. They will learn to trust you and feel like a responsible member of the team as they close doors and hold handrails themselves. Even those who have not yet undergone training will feel more comfortable from the nonverbal and verbal clues you give and from the confident manner in which you lead them.

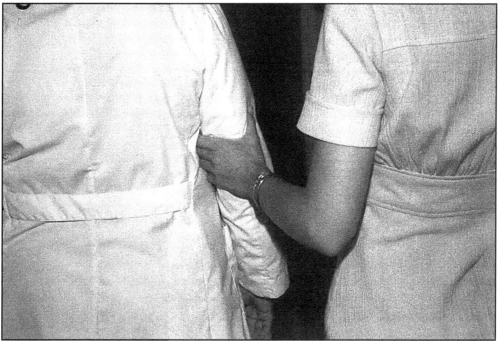

Figure 9-5. The person being guided holds the guide's arm above the elbow and walks half a pace behind.

Teachers of the Visually Impaired

Blind and low vision students have several choices of educational institutions. There are many residential schools for the blind where educational pursuits and rehabilitation are undertaken at the same center. The students live and study with other blind children. In 1976, a federal mandate, Public Law 94-142, was passed that requires public schools to provide services to all handicapped children. Since that time most residential schools have only the most severely handicapped students in residence and provide medical services as well. Since 1993, the Americans with Disabilities Act also mandated that public institutions make adaptations for persons with disabilities. This provides for a great deal of services to visually impaired students in the public schools, especially if the parents advocate for their child.

The majority of low vision and blind children attend public schools in regular classrooms. They sit close to the front of the class and, if possible, use telescopes and low vision aids to help them see. Teachers of the visually impaired are trained to deal with the special needs of these students and meet with them on a daily basis or as needed. Sometimes the teachers are itinerant, only coming to the school on a prescribed schedule. Other schools have resource rooms. These are special rooms where the student can come on a scheduled visit or just drop in. There are usually adaptive devices available in resource rooms such as CCTVs, recorded materials, and computers with adaptive software programs. Vision teachers might transfer handouts and reading assignments to large print. They also will arrange for the student to receive textbooks in a large-print, Braille, or recorded version. In addition, they might read a test to a student so it can be taken orally or transpose it into Braille.

Although it is sometimes a disadvantage to the children who need services, it is an advantage to providers of low vision care that there are usually only one or two teachers of the visually impaired in any given district. As a result, the same teachers will work with the child throughout his or her entire school career. The teachers provide continuity and a strong support to the child and the family. They will recommend low vision testing and work closely with parents, doctors, and low vision clinics to provide complete services to their students and are intimately familiar with many helpful resources. If you are going to see a low vision patient of school age, be sure to invite the vision teacher to the appointment or at least speak to the teacher by phone before and after the visit. He or she will provide very valuable information about the child's near and distance needs in the school environment.

Occupational Therapists

Occupational therapists are medical professionals who help patients adjust to any disability in order to continue performing activities of daily living and/or vocational pursuits. Although they are very well trained, they learn to deal with many different disabilities and sometimes their specific knowledge of low vision is limited. Because of this, it is better to work as a team with an occupational therapist rather than just refer a patient for services without consultation and recommendations to the therapist. Occupational therapists may work in hospitals, clinics, rehabilitation centers, or schools. Some low vision clinics have come to prefer the services of occupational therapists over those of VRTs or O&M instructors because third-party payers will cover their services. This is simply because occupational therapists are considered medical professionals while VRTs and O&M instructors are considered to be teachers.

This discrepancy might change in the near future. In 2006, The Center for Medicare and Medicaid Services implemented a 5-year project in selected areas to examine whether vision rehabilitation services should be covered by Medicare. They will also study whether Part B should cover vision rehabilitation services that are performed by "low vision therapists" under the general supervision of a physician the same way it covers those services when provided by an occupational or physical therapist.

To contact rehabilitation personnel in your area, ask the state department of blind services. Vision teachers can be located through the superintendent of school or the state department of education (usually in the special services department).

Bibliography

Scheiman M, Scheiman M, Whittaker S. *Low Vision Rehabilitation: A Practical Guide for Occupational Therapists.* Thorofare, NJ: SLACK Incorporated; 2007.

Silverstone B, Lang MA, Rosenthal B, Faye EE, eds. *The Lighthouse Handbook on Vision Impairment and Vision Rehabilitation.* New York, NY: Oxford University Press; 2000.

Chapter 10

Providing Low Vision Care in the Private Practice or Clinic

KEY POINTS

- If your office plans to provide a higher level of low vision care, extra training and more equipment will be necessary.

- It is relatively inexpensive to purchase the equipment and supplies necessary for providing basic low vision care, and the space it requires is minimal.

- Rehabilitation and referral agencies should be contacted before seeing your first patient so all necessary information and referral forms are on hand.

Levels of Care

All ophthalmology and optometry offices and clinics should be providing some form of low vision care. Patients with subnormal vision present to every office. The staff should be prepared to deal with the needs of these patients in a preplanned way so no patient in need is ever overlooked. Each office must decide what services and support it can realistically provide depending on the interests and expertise of its staff members. However, all practices can provide service at one of the following three levels of care.

Basic Level of Care

At a basic level it is only required to recognize the needs of low vision patients and be ready to refer them to appropriate agencies for the help they need. The office staff should take the time to familiarize themselves with the techniques of testing distance and near acuity in low vision patients. Every staff member who does initial patient testing should use low vision acuity testing methods on *every* patient whose vision falls below the 20/40 level. In this way, no patient will be overlooked and the method of recording acuity will be standardized. The accuracy that is ensured by using consistent testing methods will also be helpful when making referrals for other services.

Time is also required on the part of the professional staff and assistants to compile a selection of referral materials. The office should have several brochures or handouts at the ready, preprinted in large, bold type. One handout should define low vision and provide references about where patients can receive further information. Addresses, phone contacts, and web sites for the American Foundation for the Blind, the National Association for Visually Handicapped (NAVH), the National Library Service for the Blind and Physically Handicapped, and any local and state agencies should be included. Another handout should provide the name and contact information for established low vision clinics in the community. If any of these agencies require referral forms, they should be readily available at the office to be filled out and signed immediately so the transition is smooth and quick. These forms and referrals should be researched and prepared ahead of time and a stock kept handy at the front desk and in each exam room.

In the reception area or waiting room there should be a few copies of the *Reader's Digest Large Print for Easier Reading Edition* and some sample non-optical aids such as a check writing guide and a large-print watch. Usually companies that provide non-optical aids are happy to send a collection of catalogues to a medical office to be given out to patients as well.

Intermediate Level of Care

If your office or clinic staff wishes to provide some minimal low vision services on site, some actual dispensing of low vision aids occurs. Offices in this category should provide all of the same information and referral materials mentioned above in addition to separate instructions on using and maintaining the correct focal distance for each type of optical aid.

For the actual exam all that is required is a table that can accommodate a reading stand and light, reading materials, and a stock of basic low vision aids (Figure 10-1). The examination equipment is already available in most offices, although distance and near test charts modified for testing low vision will have to be ordered (Figures 10-2 and 10-3).

The staff should be trained to teach patients to use magnifiers. Knowledge of focal distance, how to hold hand magnifiers, how to use a reading stand, and the basics of appropriate illumination and light are necessary for all staff who will be working with patients. There are several

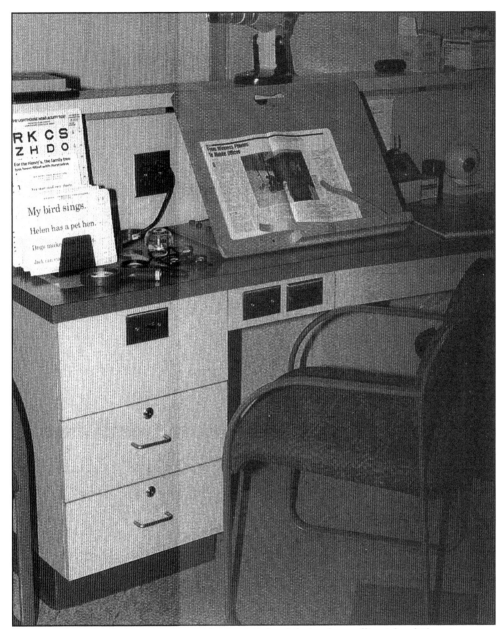

Figure 10-1. A simple low vision setup in a general ophthalmology office takes little extra space and requires a minimum of new equipment.

places for the office personnel to receive training as low vision assistants. Lighthouse International offers training both on site and online to all eyecare providers. They provide a wide array of courses appropriate for assistants, technicians, optometrists, and physicians. The Hadley School for the Blind also offers courses to professionals on low vision and blindness issues. Training and certification are also provided by the Academy for Certification of Vision Rehabilitation and Education Professionals. See the web sites list at the end of this chapter for contact information on all these programs.

Figure 10-2. Handheld distance test charts are fine for an office with a small volume of low vision patients. This distance chart is calibrated for use at 10 feet (3 meters) but can be moved closer. (Photo courtesy of Good-Lite, Elgin, IL.)

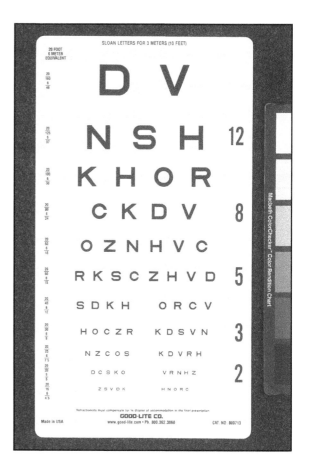

Figure 10-3. Near cards in the general office should be usable for all patients. If low vision evaluations are carried out on a daily basis, patients in need of service can be identified. (Photo courtesy of Good-Lite, Elgin, IL.)

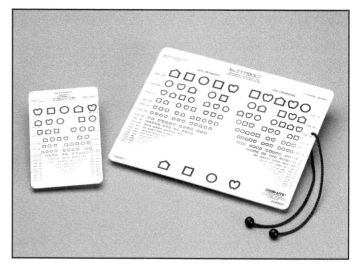

Advanced Care and Full-Service Clinics

Offices that strive to offer full-service low vision care should ensure that every person on the low vision staff is aware of the visual aids available for more severe disabilities including extensive visual field loss. All staff should also be knowledgeable of other aspects of low vision and rehabilitation. Vision rehabilitation therapists and/or occupational therapists should be hired or closely available to work with patients on adaptations to their daily living needs. Eyecare providers should become knowledgeable about bioptic telescopes, electronic equipment, and assistive technology devices. Also, the staff must be prepared to work with patients who have far more vision loss than those who just need a hand magnifier. The staff should be well versed in the services available for the blind and severely visually handicapped patient and be knowledgeable about rehabilitation centers in the area, as well as how to make appropriate referrals.

Equipment and Supplies

Whatever level of service your office decides to offer, this section will present the information necessary to get you started in providing care to your low vision patients. All offices must begin by doing research and ordering supplies. Before seeing any patients, compile the necessary stationary and office supplies. The information and addresses in this book should be enough to get you started.

Basic Level

At a minimum, every office should have the following:
- Large-print calling cards with your clinic name and phone number
- A distance test chart for low vision (see Chapter 6 for details)
- A near test chart and continuous text reading cards (see Chapter 6)
- Catalogues of suppliers of non-optical aids and some samples such as:
  - Typoscopes and check writing guides
  - Telephone dials with large-print numbers
- Referral forms for local low vision clinics that have a proven track record of competence
- Referral forms for support agencies
- Packets of informational material on low vision (see Chapter 5)

Intermediate Level

Offices that are planning to dispense magnifiers and other basic low vision aids should also have the following supplies in stock:
- Additional exam equipment such as:
  - Distance acuity log charts on an illuminated rolling stand
  - Contrast sensitivity test charts
  - A good trial frame (adult and pediatric) and lens set
  - Handheld cross cylinders of ±0.5 and ±1.00
  - Reading stand
  - Good task lighting of one or two varieties
  - Reading materials in large and small print

Figure 10-4. Several powers of magnifying spectacles should be kept on hand for low vision assessment.

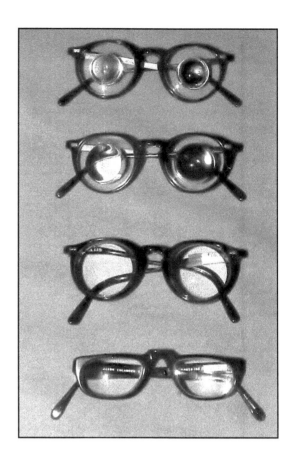

Figure 10-5. Each office should have a stock of various hand and stand magnifiers for use during examination and for lending to patients. (Photo courtesy of CTP Coil, Slough, Berkshire, UK.)

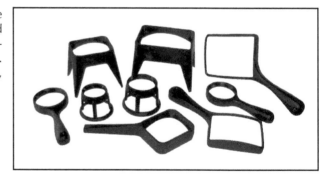

⮿ Handouts for patients on how to use the aids and maintain focal distance
⮿ Handouts for patients on spotting, scanning, and tracking as necessary with individual aids
- Optical aids in these general categories (Figures 10-4 and 10-5):
    ⮿ Handheld magnifiers of approximately 5 D, 10 D, 15 D, and 20 D
    ⮿ Folding pocket magnifiers of 10 D to 20 D
    ⮿ Stand magnifiers of approximately 10 D, 15 D, 20 D, and 25 D
    ⮿ Half-eye prismatic spectacles of 6 D, 8 D, and 10 D

      ▲ Full-frame microscopic spectacles of 4× to 10× (correction should be in both lenses as a trial pair although they will only be dispensed monocularly)

      ▲ One or two monocular telescopes in powers of 2.5× to 10×. It is best to have on hand a variety of handheld, clip-on, and head-borne binocular types

- Additional non-optical aids such as, but not limited to, the following:

      ▲ Large-print syringes and syringe magnifiers

      ▲ Large-print or talking pill containers

      ▲ Other large-print and talking medical supplies

      ▲ Check writing guides and a pack of dummy checks for practicing (these checks can be obtained from a local bank)

      ▲ A telephone with large-print buttons

      ▲ Needle threader and some spools of thread (black, white, and a neutral color)

      ▲ Large-print playing cards and one or two adapted games

      ▲ Several typoscopes (for office use during the exam and while training with aids)

      ▲ Dark Sharpie™ or 20/20™ pens (both from Sanford, Oak Brook, IL) for writing

      ▲ NoIR™ (South Lyon, MI) or SolarShield™ (Dioptics, San Luis Obispo, CA) sunglasses in several densities

Advanced Level

In order to provide full-service low vision services, offices should have all of the above as well as some or all of the following:

- A set of trial bioptic telescopic lenses
- Magnifiers and telescopes in the stronger powers and unique varieties
- A collection of loupes
- Materials to help with the training of spotting, scanning, and tracking with aids
- Adaptive software for computers, both large print and synthesized voice
- A selection of CCTVs and other electronic reading devices
- Electronic aids such as global positioning system devices, color tellers, and adaptive cell phone systems

Selecting which types of aids to stock in each of these categories is a personal choice. There are so many catalogues of aids available that it can become a considerable chore deciding which ones to purchase. Each experienced low vision provider has his or her own favorites to recommend, so talk to someone who is already in low vision practice for advice. Alternatively, several companies market starter kits. Designs for Vision (Ronkonkoma, NY) offers several of these starter kits including the option of renting one for a daily fee. Many offices may prefer the rental option to evaluate the types of aids they wish to have in their office collection before purchasing. Designs for Vision trial kits primarily include spectacles (half eye, microscopic, and telescopic) and bioptics. Several kits also include distance and near test charts and a carrying case. For the more basic aids such as hand and stand magnifiers and loupes in addition to bioptics and telescopes, Eschenbach Optik of America (Ridgefield, CT) and S. Walters (Agoura Hills, CA) also offer some good starter kits and display cases. Each of these companies only market their own brand of magnifiers, so contact some of the other suppliers as well to see if they will offer rental options or starter kits.

If you would like more flexibility, your office can order aids individually. Each company has several classic aids and designs that are excellent and have not been reproduced by other companies. In addition to those already mentioned, Selsi (Midland Park, NJ) makes excellent and inexpensive telescopes, and CTP Coil (Slough, Berkshire, UK) makes some very good stand magnifiers. So try not to limit your options to one or two companies before you assess several others and find the aids that will become favorites for you and your patients. There are several clearinghouses, such as the NAVH Low Vision Service and Independent Living Aids, that market optical and non-optical aids from many different manufacturers.

However you stock your office with optical and non-optical low vision aids, it is a good idea to order more than one of each type. That way you will have one for demonstration in the office and at least one to lend or dispense to patients who find it helpful. If you can send an aid home with a patient on the first visit, it is far more positive than to order one and make the patient wait for it to arrive. If you lend the aid, the patient can use it immediately and try it in the home or work setting before his or her own is ordered. That way, any problems can be identified before the aid is purchased. This allows the patient to be more honest about difficulties and therefore more successful in the long run. Some patients need to try several aids before finding the one that is a good fit and satisfactory for individual needs.

There are several options when choosing a distance acuity test chart. For the office that is not going to be doing much low vision work, the handheld charts are fine. There are many varieties to choose from (see Chapter 6 on Assessment of Visual Function) including the HOTV test chart and the Sloan letters test chart. The Feinbloom Distance Test Chart for the Partially Sighted is a commonly used, simple flip chart that also comes in a pediatric version. For more sophisticated low vision acuity testing, logMAR tests such as the Ferris-Bailey ETDRS acuity test chart are preferred. The Lighthouse Distance Visual Acuity Test version attaches to a rolling cart specifically designed for low vision so that it can be moved to nearer testing distances and also illuminated from behind. It is labeled with logMAR, Sloan, and Snellen acuity notations. All of these charts are simple to use, logically designed, and have helpful conversions for different testing distances. There are also versions of these charts for use by pediatric or non-English-speaking patients. The HOTV test comes with an accompanying card so that the letter viewed at distance can be located and pointed to on the near card.

A set of continuous text cards for adults and one for children is mandatory equipment to assess functional near acuity with low vision aids. Sets should be available in all languages spoken by a large number of patients who visit the office. Near vision can also be tested using MN Read or logMAR reading cards which are well calibrated for near use. Every office that intends to provide low vision services should have at least one version of the near testing cards.

Your office will also need a reading stand and appropriate task lighting. For lamps, have a couple varieties of good quality desk lamps. Each should have a flexible arm and a heavy base so it will not fall over. It should have a rounded shade or other method of directing the light to the page. Plastic shades are preferred over metal so that the user is not burned when close to the lamp. The office should also maintain a stock of bulbs for use in the reading lamp. Sixty-watt incandescent bulbs or the lower-watt, energy-efficient, fluorescent light bulbs are best. These low energy bulbs are cooler and safer than the incandescent as long as your patient is not bothered by the fluorescence, which many are not.

The reading materials (Figure 10-6) that should be on hand for near testing should include:
- A large-print book or *Reader's Digest*
- *Time* or other newsmagazine (black print on glossy white pages)

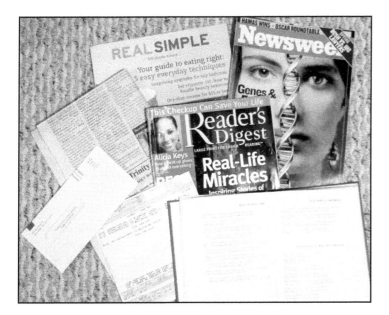

Figure 10-6. Have several types of reading materials on hand so acuity can be assessed using real-life situations.

- Newspaper front page (less contrast to the print than a newsmagazine)
- Newspaper obituary page (smaller print and of high importance to elderly patients)
- Sports, cooking, travel, and other specialty magazines
- A piece of correspondence such as a utility bill or credit card statement
- A Bible in regular size print and one in large print
- A supply of children's books and comics

Finding Referral Agencies

Before your clinic services its first low vision patient, locate your state agency for the blind and familiarize yourself with the laws governing care to the visually impaired in your state. You can find your state agency by contacting the National Council of State Agencies for the Blind at their web site (www.ncsab.org) and clicking on the directory link. By contacting the state agency that oversees care to the blind, you will be directed to several other sources for blind and low vision care in your area. Each one leads to others and soon you will have a good library of local resources. On your first contact, ask about services for children as well as services for working adults and seniors. Find the name of several low vision clinics and rehabilitation centers in your area and go visit them. Make an appointment with a rehabilitation counselor to ask questions about state and federal help and regulations and the levels of service for low vision patients who are not legally blind. For each contact, also determine how to make referrals and request copies of all necessary forms.

If your office is only going to provide information and referrals, you will need to become familiar with all of the low vision clinics in your area and choose the one or two where you would most like to refer patients. Contact and visit each office that offers low vision care and do not limit yourself to just ophthalmology or just optometry. There are excellent low vision clinics in both settings and many full-service clinics have both specialties on staff. Although some offices advertise low vision care, they might actually only have one or two aids in stock and have minimal experience. Others will be full-service low vision clinics and you cannot tell until you visit them on site. Likewise, if you are in an optometry office, do not assume that the local ophthalmology clinic has well-established low vision services. Look for the low vision clinic that will offer the best services and follow-up to your patients. If it is somewhat of a distance away, have a second choice closer to home in case your patients are not willing or are unable to travel.

Involving the Community

There are many possibilities for low vision clinics to become vital players in the local community, bringing together diverse groups with interests in low vision. By inviting vision teachers to the evaluation of their students you will become involved in the schools. Libraries are always receptive to new materials and would appreciate information on where to send for books and periodicals pertaining to low vision. Civic organizations such as Lions Clubs like to have guest speakers, and those interested in eyecare are always welcome. A discussion of the services your low vision clinic provides will go a long way to bringing in more patients and will result in heightened community support and referrals. The Lions Club is also known for funding special programs for vision care and may become involved in helping to establish your clinic or some of its programs.

If your clinic or office is in a small community, you may be the only resource for many people who have been looking for help. You can become a clearinghouse for information or even create a support group for local families who have a relative with low vision. In one community, a local support group evolved from just such an effort. Local teachers, low vision providers, rehabilitation personnel, and families with low vision children began to meet monthly. The first half hour was spent mingling and talking and sharing stories. Then a speaker from an agency or organization would talk for a half hour, followed by refreshments and more mingling. It was sometimes difficult to get the families to leave because they shared so much in common and had been experiencing it alone for so long. It took very little effort on the part of the organizers and brought together diverse parts of the community with common interests. Be creative in your own area and you never know what might evolve.

A simpler way to provide services to your patients is to organize a monthly meeting of patients with similar diagnoses. This can be in your office or in a public setting. There is no need for a specific group leader, although you may give a talk on the disease process and take questions. Mostly, it will be to allow time for patients with similar experiences to share time and stories with one another. The best support for someone in need is the companionship of other people with a similar challenge. They support each other emotionally and share information about agencies or supplies they have found to be helpful.

Helpful Web Sites

Vision Test Charts
- **Good-Lite**
  www.good-lite.com

Reading Stands

- **American Printing House for the Blind**
  www.aph.org
- **Dynamic Living**
  www.dynamic-living.com/book_stand1.html
- **Levenger**
  www.levenger.com

(Most all of the non-optical aid catalogues also carry reading stands.)

Education, Training, and Certification of Staff

- **Academy for Certification of Vision Rehabilitation and Education Professionals**
  www.acvrep.org/Low_Vision
- **Hadley School for the Blind**
  www.hadley-school.org
- **Lighthouse International**
  www.lighthouse.org/about/education/programs.htm

For web sites of vendors of low vision aids, see:
- Optical aids—end of Chapter 2
- Non-optical and daily living aids—end of Chapter 3
- Electronic aids and assistive technology—end of Chapter 4
- More exam equipment, lighting, and reading stands—end of Chapters 3 and 6

Bibliography

Faye EE, Albert DL, Freed B, Seidman KR, Fischer M. *The Lighthouse Ophthalmology Resident Training Manual: A New Look at Low Vision Care.* New York, NY: Lighthouse International; 2000.

Chapter 11

Case Histories

KEY POINTS

- Be careful not to "pigeonhole" your patients into particular groups. Each patient, even among those with the same diagnosis, will have unique individual needs. The low vision provider's challenge is to *understand* each of these needs and offer as much assistance and support as possible.

- Patients' needs can be met in the low vision clinic or through referral.

- Offer but do not force suggestions on patients who are resistant to them. Remember that success or failure depends largely on each individual's personality and the level of acceptance of his or her visual loss.

The various parts of a low vision examination have been covered in previous chapters of this book. Each part of the examination and referral procedure was treated separately. In actual practice, however, the examination is a cohesive unit, not the sum of individual unrelated tests. The following cases are presented to illustrate how several extensive low vision evaluations might flow. Each represents someone who has been seen in low vision clinics and rehabilitation centers. Following these patients along through their low vision visit should help you get a feel for how to approach the individuals who will come for low vision care. In reading the case histories, remember that the suggestions given are just that. They are only suggestions. For each patient, there may be many right answers. Whatever choice is made, if the individual is able to accomplish his or her goals, the low vision visit has been a success.

These case histories depict extensive or unusual low vision cases. Try to remember, however, that low vision care is a part of a "normal" patient examination as well. Test distance acuity at closer distances, test near acuity with continuous text reading cards, and use the modified refractometry techniques of low vision for any patient whose vision falls below the 20/50 level even temporarily. You will always have a more accurate assessment of vision if you do so. Test for near reading adds with +2.50 lenses in a trial frame and continuous text reading cards at 40 cm for any patient with a need for bifocal power greater than +3.00 D. Keep in mind the information on psychology of visual loss for all patients, even those who are simply postoperative cataract patients. These techniques can and should be used routinely. When low vision care becomes a part of normal patient management, the extra help needed by the more severely impaired patients will become second nature. Only then will we be providing optimum care to all patients.

Case One: Woman with Macular Degeneration

History:

Delores is a 72-year-old woman with bilateral intraocular lenses and macular degeneration OU. She had laser treatment OS 1 year ago and the vision has remained stable.

Social History:

Delores is a widow who came to the exam alone via senior bus from a local assisted living center. She takes her meals in a common dining room at the center. A maid is provided, who comes once a week to vacuum, dust, change the bed linens, and clean the bathroom. Delores also has access to the services of visiting nurses and other therapists as needed for medical or self-care.

Goals and Visual Needs:

Delores has been only a moderate reader all her life. She enjoyed reading magazines and occasionally the daily newspaper. Since her vision has deteriorated she misses reading and writing letters to her family. She would like to be able to read her mail, the obituaries in the newspaper, and her Bible.

Observations:

During the discussion and exam Delores talks mainly about missing her family and being alone. She adjusts well to near reading distances, but becomes distracted easily. It is difficult to decide if she will remember much of what you tell her. General frailty and weakness cause her to have a slight hand tremor.

Distance Acuity with Current Rx:
OD: +1.00 -2.75 x 170 10/80 (20/160 equivalent)
OS: +1.75 -2.00 x 006 10/400 (20/800 equivalent)

Near Acuity:
OU: 3M+ at 33 cm with current +3.00 adds

Refraction in Trial Frame:
OD: +0.75 -2.00 x 170 (visual acuity 10/70)   Near with +2.50 adds @ 40 cm 3M+
OS: +1.75 -3.25 x 005 (visual acuity 10/400)   Near vision too poor to consider

Near Test (with +2.50 adds at 40 cm reading distance):
OU: 3M+ print can be read (so acuity is 40/3M or 40 cm/300 cm)
$300 \div 40 = 7.50$, so a +7.50 reading add should be tried

Trials with Low Vision Aids:
- *Spectacles with Near Rx:* +8.25 -2.00 x 165, visual acuity is 1.5M, 1M if the paper is steadied.
- *Hand Magnifier (8 D):* Difficulty: She is unable to use it due to hand weakness and tremor.
- *Stand Magnifier (9 D):* With current bifocal and the stand magnifier she reads 1M print. Difficulty: It slides down the page and she loses her place easily.

Other Tests:
- Decreased contrast sensitivity
- Central scotoma at near on Amsler grid testing, but the test was unreliable so indefinite

Low Vision Recommendations

Reading Spectacles:
- OD +8.25 -2.00 x 165 (distance Rx with +7.50 for near).
- These would be for general use and reading large print.
- The vision OS is poor enough for just a balance correction and no base-in prism is needed for binocularity.
- If she experiences annoying blur, the left eye can be fogged or occluded.
- Work carefully with Delores to teach her the closer reading distance (13.3 cm, which is approximately 5 inches). This will take practice on her part.

Stand Magnifier:
- Try a 5 D bright field globe magnifier (Figure 11-1) for use with her low vision reading glasses.
- Good for reading obituaries, phone book listings, and other small print. (Usually if someone can read 1.5M with glasses, this is just enough to allow reading 1M print.) There are several types, and some are heavy. Suggest a lighter weight variety so it does not slide down a reading stand and is easier for her to handle.

Figure 11-1. A bright field stand magnifier is very easy to use for short-term reading, and good hand strength is not necessary since it sits on the page.

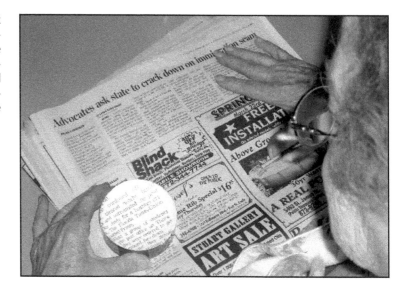

- Work with her to be able to move the magnifier across reading material and maintain her place on the page.

Non-Optical Aids:

Lighting:
- Patients with macular degeneration react well to improved illumination, so recommend appropriate task lighting.
- Teach Delores to position light correctly for optimum illumination without shadow.

Reading Stand:
- A reading stand will help hold the material still and maintain a constant reading distance, eliminating some of the problem caused by her hand tremor.
- Set the stand for a 13.3 cm reading distance in a position to relieve back and neck strain.

Writing Aids:
- Delores likes to correspond with her family by mail. Recommend a check writing guide, a typoscope, and an envelope writing guide. Bold lined paper may be helpful as well.
- A black felt tip marker (20/20 pen™) will help her see her own writing better; suggest that family members use one as well when they write to her.

Large-Print and Recorded Material:
- Delores is only a moderate reader, so does not need a great deal of reading material.
- She would probably appreciate a large-print Bible and large-print magazines such as *Reader's Digest*. Give her the addresses of vendors for these items.
- Sign her up as a member of the National Association of Visually Handicapped (NAVH). They will send information on vision loss, and they offer a large-print lending library if she chooses to read more.
- A referral to the National Library Service for the Blind and Physically Handicapped (NLS) will provide access to recorded books and periodicals.

Electronic Aids:
- Delores is a good candidate for a CCTV.
- If she cannot afford one, perhaps the assisted living center could purchase one for use by all residents. This would provide assistance with reading mail independently, looking at photographs of the family, and reading magazines or obituaries.

Support Services:
- Find out which professional service providers are available on staff at the assisted living center.
- If there is an occupational therapist, suggest a home visit to mark any dials or switches with large-print labels or bump-ons.
- If there is a social worker, request that a friend, family member, or staff member help Delores with the use of optical aids, lighting, and a reading stand in her home setting.
- Delores will need follow-up support at home to experience success and learn how to adjust the lighting for her personal reading and writing needs.
- Also discuss isolation issues with the social worker. Ask if anything can be done to increase social contact for Delores. If she is not sociable at the assisted living facility, perhaps she would prefer to be involved at her senior center, house of worship, or other organization.
- A volunteer may be found who will read to her several times per week. This person could help read mail or the newspaper and also provide companionship.

Follow-Up:
- Order the magnifiers, reading stand, and lamp or provide them from your office stock. Your office could also order the large-print Bible and *Reader's Digest*. Delores will find it difficult to do so herself, and these items would likely go unordered.
- Schedule a follow-up in 1 to 3 weeks to evaluate her success at home with her low vision aids. A helper should be along for this session.
- Provide lessons to Delores and to her helper as well as preprinted instructions in large print on maintaining focal distances, tracking with the magnifier, and using task lighting. She will need more than one follow-up visit. Since she is easily distracted and lonely, she may not be motivated to practice at home.

Case Two: Middle-Aged Man with Proliferative Diabetic Retinopathy

History:

Marc is a 46-year-old man with proliferative diabetic retinopathy. He has undergone laser treatment multiple times in each eye. His visual loss has remained stable for over a year, but his acuity fluctuates daily. His diabetes is treated with insulin, but is not well controlled. Adjustments are made often because his blood sugar varies frequently. He has some peripheral neuropathy and experiences trouble walking. He has had to quit his profession as an electrician as a result of the visual and physical disabilities. He would like to return to work. He has also given up driving since his vision dropped below legal limits. He is sensitive to light and wears sunglasses at all times, sometimes even indoors.

Social History:

Marc lives with his wife, who does the majority of the cooking, cleaning, and driving. He enjoys lifting weights for exercise and has an extensive coin collection. Emotionally, he is well-adjusted to his disability with realistic expectations and a good support network. He understands that his vision and his diabetes may worsen, but would like to return to work or try aids that will help him regain some independence. He is motivated to attempt anything that will help.

Goals and Visual Needs:

Marc would like to see well enough to return to work. If he cannot do the duties of an electrician, he is willing to learn a new trade or profession. He would like to be able to drive again and to be more helpful with household chores to take some burden off his wife. He would also like to enjoy his coin collection and perhaps start a side business buying and selling coins on eBay™ or another Internet site.

Observations:

Marc is intelligent and motivated, yet realistic about his physical limitations. He listens well and is willing to experiment with any aids and techniques that might assist in reaching his goals.

Distance Acuity with Current Rx:
OD: +1.25 -0.50 x 072 (20/70)
OS: +0.75 -0.75 x 105 (20/50-)

Near Acuity:
OD: 2.5M with current Rx and no add
OS: 2.5M less well with current Rx and no add

Refraction in Trial Frame:
OD: +1.00 -0.75 x 075 (20/70+)
OS: +1.00 -0.75 x 105 (20/50-)

Near Test (with +2.50 adds over Rx at 40 cm):
1.5M print can be read (so near acuity is 40/1.5M or 40 cm/150 cm)
$150 \div 40 = 3.75$, so a +3.75 reading add should be tried

Trials with Low Vision Aids:
Spectacles: With +3.75 adds he reads 1M easily

Other Tests:
- Moderately decreased contrast sensitivity
- Decreased acuity with glare testing
- Amsler grid shows multiple random scotomas just outside the macular area

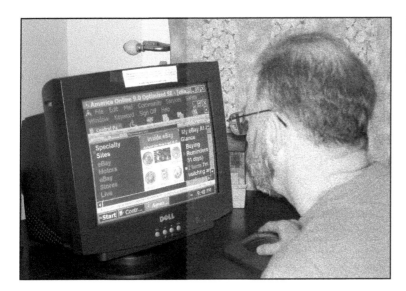

Figure 11-2. Computer accessibility options help provide visual access to the Internet.

Low Vision Recommendations

Spectacles:
- Provide a +3.75 add with his new Rx.
- The lenses in his glasses can be tinted to help with glare and photosensitivity. Write a recommendation on the Rx for light-absorbing lenses.

Stand Magnifier:

Try a 10 or 12 D stand magnifier for viewing his coin collection. (The extra power is for the tiny dates and markings on coins.) An illuminated magnifier may be too bright, or it might help to reduce the glare from task lighting. Experiment with both types.

Bioptics:

Marc should consider bioptic telescopes for driving. Refer him to an established low vision clinic with experience prescribing these.

Non-Optical Aids:
Lighting:
- Most task lighting will probably be too bright for Marc and cause him discomfort.
- Ordinary room light or task lighting at a distance further from the reading material will be more efficient.
- A diffuser or filter over the lampshade may help as well.
- Yellow sunglasses or filters to increase contrast may help under lower light conditions.

Electronic Aids:
- Marc is an excellent candidate for adaptive computer programs (Figure 11-2). Enlarging the print on his computer and a change in polarity to white letters on a dark background will be helpful. A program such as ZoomText would allow him to read email and access the Internet, including eBay™.

Other Non-Optical Aids:
- Marc would be helped by a syringe magnifier and other medical supplies to help him with his blood sugar testing and insulin administration.
- He can order labels for kitchen appliances and adaptive tools to help with cooking and cleaning.
- He will benefit from a large-print or talking watch and calculator. Provide him with a catalogue of some major suppliers, such as LS&S and Independent Living Aids.

Support Services:
- Provide him with a list of web sites that will direct him to support groups and information on low vision and on diabetic eye disease.
- Marc is a candidate for vocational training. Refer him to the state office of vocational rehabilitation or blindness services. A rehabilitation counselor will evaluate Marc, recommend appropriate training programs, and defray the costs of most low vision aids if he is eligible for services and if the aids assist him in becoming re-employed.
- His acuity is not at the level of legal blindness. Therefore he might not be immediately eligible for services, but might be accepted due to his other disabilities and medical needs. In view of his young age, motivation, and employability, refer him now and let the state agency make the determination of eligibility.

Follow-Up:
- Schedule a 1- to 2-week follow-up appointment.
- Determine if he is experiencing success with his tinted glasses and high power reading adds.
- Evaluate his lighting needs further. Question if the suggested lighting is helpful or if there are any further difficulties.
- Follow up on any referrals you made to make sure he has appointments for other services.

Case Three: Child with Ocular Albinism

History:
Claire is a 6-year-old girl with ocular albinism. She in in first grade and was referred from her elementary school nurse, who did not send any particular recommendations or list of concerns and is not present at the exam. Claire's parents do not think she needs any help because she is functioning as well as a sighted child. She has had regular eye exams since birth and her vision is stable and without pathology other than the albinism. Her ophthalmologist has mentioned that she might need visual assistance in the future, but has never referred her for a low vision exam.

Social History:
Claire is the middle child of three. Her older brother is a bright child in fourth grade, and she has a 2-year-old sister. Claire is the only one with ocular albinism. She plays normally with her siblings and is extremely well adjusted. She can run and play with other children, see small details, and is progressing in reading.

Goals and Visual Needs:

Claire is not aware of her visual loss as a disability. She has functioned well and does not know if she wants any magnifiers or optical help. The parents are interested to learn of any recommendations, but they do not feel the need for any intervention at this point in time. Since the teacher is not present the educational goals are not definite.

Observations:

Claire is a lively young girl, normal in appearance. She maintains some pigment in her skin and hair. She has nystagmus and a clear lack of pigment in both irises.

Distance Acuity with Current Rx:

OD: 10/100 with no correction (20/200 equivalent)
OS: 10/70 with no correction (20/140 equivalent)

Near Acuity:

OU: 1M print easily without correction (by holding the reading material at an approximately 6-inch distance from her eyes)

Refraction in Trial Frame:

(Note: It is especially important that Claire's refraction be done in a trial frame because of the presence of nystagmus. The larger field of view will allow her to see better than through the small aperture of a phoropter. It also allows for more accurate retinoscopy.)
OD: -0.50 -2.00 x 167 (10/70)
OS: -0.75 sphere (10/60)

Near Test (+2.50 adds over Rx at a 40 cm):

OU: 3M with both eyes (so near acuity is 40/2.5M or 40 cm/250 cm)
250 ÷ 40 = 6.25, so a 6.25 reading add would be the power of choice

Low Vision Recommendations

Optical Aids:

None Necessary for Near:

- Claire has an accommodative amplitude large enough to supply the necessary 6.25 reading power at near without fatigue. Also, she is myopic which supplies additional plus power at near. No near correction is necessary for reading at this time.
- Mention to her parents that print size will become smaller in the higher grades and that she will lose her ability to focus at near as she grows older. She will eventually need glasses or a magnifier for near use (Figure 11-3), so she should be reevaluated at the start of each school year.

Distance Aids:

- Claire's vision improved enough with refraction to recommend glasses for distance.
- Contact lenses are helpful for patients with nystagmus, and a tinted variety could be ordered to help with photosensitivity. Discuss the possibility with her parents.

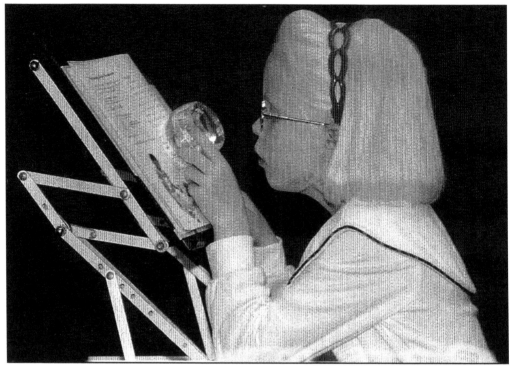

Figure 11-3. A reading stand holds material at a proper angle for use with magnifiers.

- First graders often cannot simply walk up to a distant object (such as the blackboard) as easily as when at home or in kindergarten, so a monocular handheld telescope of low power would be an excellent recommendation.
- Telescopes require several new skills such as spotting, tracking, focusing, and steadying. Claire will need several lessons from a low vision or occupational therapist to perfect her ability to use it successfully.
- Eventually Claire will be a good candidate for bioptic telescopic glasses. Refer her now to a low vision clinic that fits bioptics to get recommendations about what cues to look for to know when the time might be appropriate for their use.

Non-Optical Aids:

Lighting:
- Patients with ocular albinism are very sensitive to light. Normal lighting is often too bright so absorptive lenses and filters in glasses are helpful. However, albinos sometimes notice decreased visual acuity when wearing normal sunglasses, so the tint should not be too strong. NoIR Medical Technologies offers special sunglasses for albinism and have frames in adult and children's sizes.
- When reading, normal room light will be sufficient and a stronger power task lighting will probably not be necessary.
- A yellow filter to increase contrast could be tried for near work.

Electronic Aids:

- Claire sees well at near. She is not a candidate for a CCTV or other electronic magnification system yet. Recommend it to the parents for future consideration. Refer the family to some of the larger manufacturers by giving them the address, phone number, and web addresses.
- Claire will eventually experience difficulty with computer use because of the enforced longer working distance to the screen. She should already try the accessibility options on the operating system she uses to enlarge the print size and reverse polarity for glare control. The family can also consider one of the large-print programs, such as ZoomText, which allows greater flexibility in navigating through documents.
- She would also benefit from a Key to Access, a small portable flashdrive that can be loaded with accessible software and then plugged into the USB port of any computer. This would enable Claire to use her large-print software program at home, school, library, and homes of friends.
- Also recommend some large-print high contrast keyboard stickers. They are available with black print on yellow background or with white on black.

Support Services:

- Although Claire is doing very well at the moment, it is not long before she will need more assistance at school. A recommendation should be made to the school for her to receive assistance through the department of education. The school is required by law to provide her with any services or adaptive appliances necessary for her education. This includes low vision aids, electronic devices, and any educational services that would help, such as large-print textbooks and special education teachers.
- Refer the family to the National Organization for Albinism and Hypopigmentation (NOAH) at www.albinism.org. This national organization offers information and support materials as well as recommendations for the future and for social adjustment. Children with ocular albinism sometimes experience social difficulties from trying to "hide" their disability. NOAH can recommend help to the family for dealing with these emotional issues. The organization also makes recommendations for educational needs.

Follow-Up:

- Claire should return for low vision evaluation annually. As she grows up and her near demands increase, her need for magnification and electronic devices will also increase.
- Since her parents are reluctant at this time to accept the need for any intervention, they should be encouraged to make decisions annually about her changing visual needs.

Case Four: Woman with Macular Degeneration

History:

Terry is a 64-year-old woman with macular degeneration. In the past, she visited a low vision clinic and was successfully prescribed 8 D half-eye spectacles. Now she complains that she can no longer see as well with them. She says she can see better sometimes with no near correction at all.

Social History:

Terry does not work outside the home, but is involved with many civic organizations and activities. Her husband drives and takes care of the family finances, and they share the household duties. She is very intelligent and an avid reader. She has belonged to several book clubs in her community, but has not been able to read the assigned books in the past few months so has not been attending. Cooking and cleaning are not a problem to her, but she cannot read price tags while shopping.

Goals and Visual Needs:

Terry wants to be able to continue reading books for pleasure and to return to her book clubs. She also wants to be able to perform well at her civic organizations and take on more responsibility than she has been able to handle with her visual loss.

Observations:

She is a lovely older woman with a lively personality and enthusiasm. She is willing to try anything to see better. She has been very successful with low vision aids in the past and understands the changes she must make to her reading distance and perhaps to her type of lighting.

Distance Acuity with Current Rx:

OD: -2.25 sphere 10/120 (20/240 equivalent)

OS: -2.00 -0.50 x 075 10/160 (20/320 equivalent)

During acuity testing she states that she can see some of the small titles on the test better than "those huge numbers." An attempt is made to recheck the acuity with smaller optotypes because sometimes there is a minimal area of intact retina which will allow better resolution of an image than in the surrounding compromised retina.

Distance Acuity Test (using smaller characters):

OD: 10/20+ (this is a 20/40 equivalent)

OS: 10/160 (no change)

Near Acuity (with current +12 spectacles):

OD: 2.5M

OS: 3M

Refraction in Trial Frame:

OD: -2.00 -0.75 x 163 (10/120 fluently, 10/20+ reading one letter at a time)

OS: -2.25 -1.25 x 075 (10/120-)

Near Evaluation (+2.50 adds at 40 cm):

OD: with a slight eccentric viewing position, 1.5M print; so acuity is 40/1.5M or 40 cm/ 150 cm

    $150 \div 40 = 3.78$ so a 3.75 add is appropriate

Trial with Low Vision Aids:

Trial with +3.75 Adds: 1.5M- but less well because she sees fewer letters. She preferred the +2.50 add used during the evaluation.

Visual Field Evaluation:

The visual field assessment is especially important in this patient to determine the number and size of the areas of useful vision in the macular area.

Tangent Screen: Intact peripheral fields in both eyes, central scotomas OU

Amsler Grid: Central scotomas OU, but a small parafoveal area remains without distortion OD

Low Vision Recommendations

Terry prefers to read with her small area of intact macula rather than with magnification, which enlarges images outside the limits of her small usable field of view. Since the larger images are viewed with peripheral retina, she notices a decrease in the quality of her vision with magnification.

Spectacles:

- Since her low vision refractometric measurement has a -2.50 spherical equivalent, a +2.50 add renders her near prescription essentially plano for the 40 cm distance. If she notes a subjective improvement from the cylinder correction, reading glasses can be suggested.
- Encourage her to read using her area of best vision by providing eccentric viewing training.
- Advise her that the vision she has will not be destroyed by use.
- She has already used strong reading spectacles so understands the need for a close working distance. She will adapt more easily if she eventually loses more of her macular function.

Stand Magnifier:

A low power (4 to 5 D) stand magnifier will help with the reading of very small print, enlarging it to the 1.5M size that she sees well.

Bioptic Telescopes:

Refer Terry to a low vision clinic that fits bioptic telescopes. She should be evaluated because they will probably improve her distance vision to a more useful level.

Non-Optical Aids:

Lighting:

Recommend task lighting for reading indoors and a penlight or 5 D lighted hand magnifier for reading price tags in stores.

Large-Print and Recorded Books:

Although Terry can read well with her right eye, she will become fatigued when trying to read for a long time. She might enjoy listening to books on tape as well as reading. A referral to the NLS would provide her access to thousands of titles. The NAVH also has a lending library as does Bookshare.org.

Household and Daily Living Aid Items:

Since Terry is still very much involved in the keeping of her own home, she could benefit by the use of some adaptive devices. Provide her with a catalogue of products from a distributor such as Independent Living Aids. She will be able to order large-print watches and telephones, items to help in the kitchen such as a liquid level indicator so she does not overfill coffee cups, and

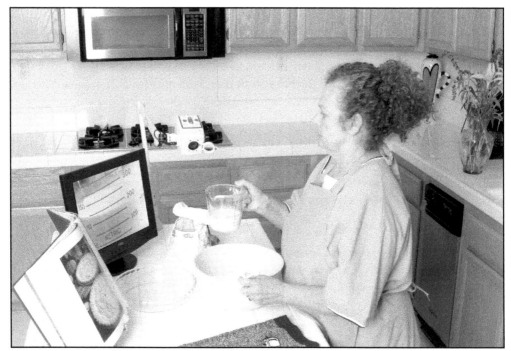

Figure 11-4. A portable CCTV can be used for cooking. Here, the level of liquid is being measured in the cup. (Photo courtesy of Enhanced Vision, Huntington Beach, CA.)

special knives that control the size of slices and protect the fingers. She might also be interested in materials to help with record keeping and finances or large-print playing cards and games. If she has the catalogue she can order whatever she likes.

Electronic Aids:
- A video reading machine would be a good choice for Terry.
- A CCTV would allow her to view photographs, maps, and any other printed material. Terry could use one for cooking (Figure 11-4) and correspondence as well. She is a good candidate for a portable model because she could attach it to her computer to magnify the words she is typing when working on her volunteer projects, take it along to meetings to make presentations, and view other speakers in the distance.
- A handheld electronic magnifier (Figure 11-5) would be helpful for shopping or any project outside the home that only requires quick checking.

Support Services:
- Not everyone is interested in joining a support group, but Terry is very likely to prefer one. Since she has a history of being involved in civic groups and book clubs already, she obviously enjoys the social contact. Referrals to the NAVH, American Council of the Blind, and the National Federation of the Blind would introduce her to the many organizations available nationwide and locally.
- She should be referred to the state agency governing blindness services since her vision falls into the category of legal blindness. In spite of the small area of good usable vision she retains, her actual visual acuity level is 20/240 OD and 20/320 OS

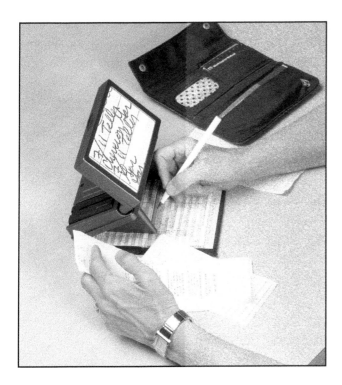

Figure 11-5. A handheld electronic magnifier has uses in and outside the home and can be carried easily in a coat pocket or purse. Some can be used for writing as well as reading. (Photo courtesy of Enhanced Vision, Huntington Beach, CA.)

(recorded at the initial exam). The agency professionals will see that she is evaluated for any other appropriate services such as occupational therapy or other rehabilitation needs.

- Terry might also offer her support to your office. With her energy and interest in civic organizations she will be a valuable volunteer. She could be very instrumental in setting up an outreach service to visually impaired patients in your office.

Case Five: Older Gentleman with Glaucoma

History:

Rob is a 78-year-old man with glaucoma. His left eye is totally blind from a central retinal vein occlusion and neovascular glaucoma. One year ago he underwent cataract extraction with intraocular lens in the right eye, but suffered some complications including elevated intraocular pressure. His vision has remained stable for 6 months.

Social History:

Rob lives with his wife, who is with him at the exam. She does all the household chores. Although he used to be the one to take care of all the financial business he is no longer able to see well enough, and his wife has taken over that responsibility as well. He is unable to read his own mail or balance his checkbook.

Goals and Visual Needs:

Rob has always been very active. He likes to boat but has to have someone along with him when he goes. He likes to fish but can no longer tie hooks. He was always outdoors and physically active, but lately has been spending time watching TV in the house.

Observations:

Rob appears depressed and poorly motivated. His wife says that he is very discouraged and thinks that nothing will help him. He seems to feel that his productive life has ended.

Distance Acuity with Current Rx:

OD: -1.00 -1.75 x 100 10/40 (20/80 equivalent)
OS: Balance Rx with no light perception

Near Acuity:

OD: 2M with current 3.50 add
OS: No light perception

Refraction in Trial Frame:

OD: -1.50 -1.50 x 105 10/30- (approximately 20/70 equivalent)
OS: Not attempted

Near Test (with +2.50 adds at 40 cm):

1.5M (acuity is 40/1.5M or 40 cm/150 cm)
150 ÷ 40 = 3.75 so a +3.75 add should be tried

Trials with Low Vision Aids:

Spectacles: Using +2.25 -1.50 x 105 for near he reads 1.5M. This is equivalent to his distance Rx with a +3.75 add. Rob is able to see well, but doesn't like the nearer reading distance.

Hand Magnifier: With distance correction and a 5 D hand magnifier he reads 1M print but complains about having to maintain the steady focal distance.

Stand Magnifier: With his current near Rx and a 5 D stand magnifier he is also able to read 1M print, but complains about the small field of view and trying to keep the print in view.

Loupe: With a 10 D clip-on loupe he is able to read the print of a newspaper obituary while keeping his hands free. He is unenthusiastic about how it attaches to his glasses and slightly tips them to one side.

Other Tests:

- Rob's visual field OD reveals a few small nasal scotomas and some decreased sensitivity but his field is otherwise full
- Contrast sensitivity is moderately diminished

Low Vision Recommendations

Spectacles:

Rob should receive a change in prescription for his new distance Rx and a stronger reading add. Since he was not happy with the reading distance of a +3.75 add, the near add could be a

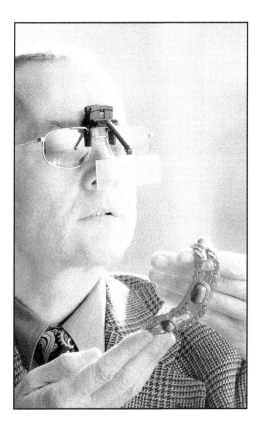

Figure 11-6. A loupe can be clipped on existing spectacles for very close work. The center clip equalizes the weight and prevents tipping of the glasses. (Photo courtesy of Eschenbach Optik of America, Ridgefield, CT.)

compromise of +3.00 or +3.25. That will be stronger than his current reading Rx but not such a drastic change to his reading habits.

Magnifiers:
A clip-on loupe of 5 to 10 D would allow Rob to attach it temporarily or flip it down when working with tying fish hooks or doing other fine work (Figure 11-6).

Non-Optical Aids:
Lighting:
Because of his decreased contrast acuity, Rob will benefit by improved lighting on his work. Recommend a task light or Ott-Lite to increase the color and contrast of his reading material.
Finance Aids:
Suggest a check writing guide, large-print checks, large-print calculator, and other materials that could help Rob regain his ability to take care of bills and correspondence. (He needs to regain a chore that makes him feel worthwhile.)

Electronic Aids:
There are probably many electronic devices that would be helpful to Rob, but it is a good idea to hold off until a follow-up visit to discuss them. He is resistant to change and might be overwhelmed by electronics at this time.

Support Services:
- Rob is discouraged and unmotivated. It is not a good idea to make many recommendations or referrals at this time. Patients like this are very difficult to predict. His discouragement may result in rejecting everything you tell him. He may not be ready to accept low vision aids for quite some time until he is over his anger and frustration and more willing to accept that his visual loss is permanent. Alternatively, he may get home and be more motivated to try his aids in private.
- Although he is complaining he cannot see, it is clear from the exam that he is actually experiencing success. He might recognize this to be true in his home setting when he can achieve some task that has been giving him difficulty.
- Provide him with an Rx for his new glasses, a 5 D stand magnifier, and a 10 D clip-on loupe to take home. Ask him to try them and come back to report about his successes and failures in 2 weeks. This will allow him to try the aids in his home environment and ensure that he returns for follow-up so you can have at least one more try.

Follow-Up:
In 2 weeks he returned for follow-up and rejected the loupes completely. He had no interest in the close working distance. He said the magnifier was okay but it did not make the print quite as dark as he would like it.

New Recommendations:
- Try a lighted 5 D magnifier instead. Work carefully with Rob and his wife on the importance of magnifier-to-page distance appropriate to a 5 D lens (20 cm).
- Again recommend a proper reading lamp.
- Suggest a pocket magnifier for use outside the home.
- Give a lot of reassurance and recommend some social service agencies and support groups in your area. It is very common for elderly patients to experience depression that goes untreated. Perhaps treating the depression will help him become more able to adjust to his visual loss. A referral to his primary care physician for evaluation could be helpful.
- Schedule another follow-up visit in 3 months. He might be more ready to accept low vision aids at that time.
- Rob will need continual reassurance. Be sure he leaves your office with a stack of reference materials, a non-optical aids catalogue, and a large-print calling card. Someday he may decide he wants help and will be able to refer to these materials.

Glossary

This book presumes that the reader has a basic understanding of optics and optical principles. Because some low vision assistants are new to the field, they may not have the background to fully understand some of the information. This is a brief description of optical principles in dictionary form to help with the comprehension of these topics. For a more thorough discussion of optics, refer to the following texts:

Lens A. *Optics, Retinoscopy, and Refractometry.* 2nd ed. Thorofare, NJ: SLACK Incorporated; 2006.
Rubin M. *Optics for Clinicians.* Gainesville, Fla: Triad Scientific Publishers; 1974.

Accommodation
Accommodation is the natural ability of the physiologic lens to change in thickness and power as a response to image distance, in order to allow that image to be focused on the retina. Closer image distances require higher powers of accommodation. The natural aging process causes accommodative ability to diminish, a process referred to as presbyopia.

Convergence
Convergence of light rays occurs when the more peripheral rays in a bundle bend inward toward the central ray or optical axis. Convergence is measured in plus diopters. Convergence does not occur "naturally." Light rays only converge after passing through a plus lens.
Convergence is also the term used to describe the turning inward of both eyes to focus on a near object.

Diopter
A diopter (D) is the unit of measurement for lenses. One diopter is the power of a lens that will focus parallel rays of light at a distance of 1 meter.

Divergence
Divergence of light rays occurs when the more peripheral rays in a bundle bend outward away from the central ray or optical axis. Divergence is measured in minus diopters. Divergence of light always occurs as light leaves its source. This might be an actual source, such as the sun or a lightbulb, or a secondary source where light is reflecting off a page or an object. As the light travels away from its source, it diverges and continues to diverge as it travels through space.

Focal Distance
Focal distance is the distance at which converging light rays come to a point of focus behind a plus lens. If the rays striking the front of a lens are parallel, the focal distance is determined by the formula $F=1/D$, where F is the focal length, 1 is 1 meter (or 100 cm), and D is the dioptric power of the lens. To determine the focal distance of a lens, divide 100 cm by the power of the lens. The result is the focal distance in centimeters.

Lens
A lens is a curved piece of glass, plastic, or other transparent material. When light rays pass through a spherical lens, the central ray passes through undeviated. Peripheral light rays are refracted, or caused to diverge or converge in relation to the central ray.

Light Rays
When light leaves its source it travels in rays. These are individual "pencils" of light that continue to travel forward undeviated in their course until affected by a lens or other refractive or reflective material. The rays travel in bundles that diverge in relation to one another.

Magnification
This refers to the enlargement in the size of an image. Magnification is measured in dioptric power or in terms of the number of times the image is enlarged, or × notation. (This book refers to magnification in diopters.)

Motion Parallax

Telescopes and other magnifiers have reduced fields of view. As an image is viewed through the small visual aperture, objects pass through the small field very quickly. This apparent motion is much faster than normal. This apparent increase in speed also occurs if the telescope itself is moved and is called motion parallax.

Optical Axis

The optical axis is the central ray of a bundle of light rays that passes through the exact center of a lens. There is no divergence or convergence. It is the ray of optimal and constant focus.

Optical Infinity

Optical infinity is the distance at which bundles of emitted light rays no longer have any measurable divergence. The light rays are referred to as being parallel, or as having "zero vergence." In reality light rays never stop diverging, but the divergence becomes too small to detect at optical infinity. In clinical optics, infinity is presumed to occur at 20 feet (or 6 meters). In geometric optics, infinity is used in its classic sense as the ultimate distance, which cannot be measured.

Prism

A prism is a lens, but is not curved. The front and back surfaces of a prism are both flat, and are arranged at an angle to each other so there is a thick end (the base) and a narrow end (the apex). Prisms cause bundles of light rays to bend in one direction instead of toward or away from the optical center. As a result images are **shifted** in the direction of the apex of the prism. One prism diopter moves an image 1 cm toward the apex of the prism at a focal distance of 1 meter. Larger displacements can be achieved by increasing the power of the prism or increasing the distance from which the object is viewed.

Refraction

Refraction is the bending of light rays by a lens. Convex (plus) lenses cause light rays to converge. Concave (minus) lenses cause light rays to diverge.

Scanning

Scanning refers to the technique of looking across a particular area by sweeping a magnifier or telescope slowly in a horizontal fashion to take in the complete field of view. It requires moving the lens, so motion parallax may interfere.

Spotting

Spotting is the technique of finding and viewing a stationary object in the field of view. Neither the eye nor the lens are moved.

Tracking

Tracking is the technique of viewing a moving object. The object and the magnifier are both in motion, so keeping them aligned can be tricky. Motion parallax and smearing of the view are common problems, as is losing the view of the object altogether.

Vergence

Vergence is the moving apart or together of light rays in a bundle. In regard to lenses, there are two vergences. First is the vergence of the rays before they strike the lens, which is dependent on distance travelled from the source. Second is the resultant vergence as the light rays leave the lens after having been refracted. The formula to determine this is $U + P = V$ where U is the unaffected vergence of the light rays just as they strike the front surface of the lens, P is the power of the lens, and V is the resultant vergence of the rays just as they leave the back surface of the lens. Vergence is measured in diopters.

Virtual Image

A virtual image appears optically to be somewhere other than its actual location.

Index

For Product Safety Concerns and Information please contact our EU
representative GPSR@taylorandfrancis.com
Taylor & Francis Verlag GmbH, Kaufingerstraße 24, 80331 München, Germany